EFFECTIVE USE OF GROUP THERAPY IN MANAGED CARE

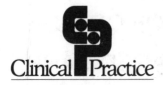

Clinical Practice

Number 29

Judith H. Gold, M.D., F.R.C.P.C.
Series Editor

EFFECTIVE USE OF GROUP THERAPY IN MANAGED CARE

Edited by

K. Roy MacKenzie, M.D., F.R.C.P.C.

Clinical Professor of Psychiatry
University of British Columbia
Vancouver, British Columbia

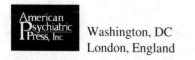

Washington, DC
London, England

Note: The authors have worked to ensure that all information in this book concerning drug dosages, schedules, and routes of administration is accurate as of the time of publication and consistent with standards set by the U.S. Food and Drug Administration and the general medical community. As medical research and practice advance, however, therapeutic standards may change. For this reason and because human and mechanical errors sometimes occur, we recommend that readers follow the advice of a physician who is directly involved in their care or the care of a member of their family.

Books published by the American Psychiatric Press, Inc., represent the views and opinions of the individual authors and do not necessarily represent the policies and opinions of the Press or the American Psychiatric Association.

Copyright © 1995 American Psychiatric Press, Inc.
ALL RIGHTS RESERVED
Manufactured in the United States of America on acid-free paper
First Edition   98   97   96   95   4   3   2   1

American Psychiatric Press, Inc.
1400 K Street, N.W., Washington, DC 20005

Library of Congress Cataloging-in-Publication Data

Effective use of group therapy in managed care / edited by K. Roy MacKenzie.
     p. cm. — (Clinical practice; no. 29)
   Includes bibliographical references and index.
   ISBN 0-88048-492-6
   1. Group psychotherapy.   2. Managed mental health care.   3. Group psychotherapy—Cost effectiveness.   I. MacKenzie, K. Roy, 1937-   .
II.   Series.
   [DNLM: 1. Psychotherapy, Group.   2. Managed Care Programs.
W1 CL767J no.29 1994 / WM 430 E27 1994]
RC488.E265   1994
616.89′152—dc20
DNLM/DLC   94-3529
for Library of Congress   CIP

British Library Cataloguing in Publication Data
A CIP record is available from the British Library.

Contents

Contributors

C. Deborah Cross, M.D.
Chair, Psychiatry Special Interest Group, American Group
Psychotherapy Association; Assistant Professor, Albany Medical
College, Director of Ambulatory Care, Albany, New York

Howard D. Kibel, M.D.
Past President, American Group Psychotherapy Association; Associate
Professor of Clinical Psychiatry, Cornell University Medical College,
The New York Hospital-Cornell Medical Center, Westchester
Division, White Plains, New York

K. Roy MacKenzie, M.D., F.R.C.P.C.
President, American Group Psychotherapy Association; Clinical
Professor of Psychiatry, University of British Columbia, Vancouver,
British Columbia

Stephen J. Melson, M.D.
Associate Professor of Psychiatry, University of Washington; Director
of Mental Health Services, Section of Psychiatry and Psychology,
Virginia Mason Medical Center, Seattle, Washington

Gerald C. Peterson, M.D.
Associate Professor of Psychiatry, Mayo Medical School; Director,
Intensive Psychotherapy Center, Mayo Clinic, Rochester, Minnesota

William E. Piper, Ph.D.
Editor, *International Journal of Group Psychotherapy,* Professor and
Co-Director of the Psychotherapy Research Centre, Department of
Psychiatry, University of Alberta, Associate Director (Program
Evaluation and Research), Division of External Psychiatric Services,
University of Alberta Hospitals, Edmonton, Alberta

Angie H. Rice, M.S.W., M.Ed.
Clinical Social Worker, East Jefferson Mental Health Center, Metairie,
Louisiana

Barry M. Segal, M.D., F.R.C.P.C.
Clinical Assistant Professor, Department of Psychiatry, University of British Columbia; Clinical Director, Psychiatric Clinics, Vancouver General Hospital, Vancouver, British Columbia

Walter N. Stone, M.D.
Past President, American Group Psychotherapy Association; Professor of Psychiatry, University of Cincinnati, Central Psychiatric Clinic, Cincinnati, Ohio

Rene Weideman, Ph.D.
Adjunct Professor, Department of Psychology, University of British Columbia; Program Coordinator, Psychiatric Clinics, Vancouver General Hospital, Vancouver, British Columbia

Introduction

to the Clinical Practice Series

Over the years of its existence the series of monographs entitled *Clinical Insights* gradually became focused on providing current, factual, and theoretical material of interest to the clinician working outside of a hospital setting. To reflect this orientation, the name of the Series has been changed to *Clinical Practice.*

The Clinical Practice Series will provide books that give the mental health clinician a practical, clinical approach to a variety of psychiatric problems. These books will provide up-to-date literature reviews and emphasize the most recent treatment methods. Thus, the publications in the Series will interest clinicians working both in psychiatry and in the other mental health professions.

Each year a number of books will be published dealing with all aspects of clinical practice. In addition, from time to time when appropriate, the publications may be revised and updated. Thus, the Series will provide quick access to relevant and important areas of psychiatric practice. Some books in the Series will be authored by a person considered to be an expert in that particular area; others will be edited by such an expert, who will also draw together other knowledgeable authors to produce a comprehensive overview of that topic.

Some of the books in the Clinical Practice Series will have their foundation in presentations at an annual meeting of the American Psychiatric Association. All will contain the most recently available information on the subjects discussed. Theoretical and scientific data will be applied to clinical situations, and case illustrations will be utilized in order to make the material even more relevant for the practitioner. Thus, the Clinical Practice Series should provide educational reading in a compact format especially designed for the mental health clinician–psychiatrist.

Judith H. Gold, M.D., F.R.C.P.C.
Series Editor

Clinical Practice Series Titles

Effective Use of Group Therapy in Managed Care (#29)
Edited by K. Roy MacKenzie, M.D., F.R.C.P.C.

Rediscovering Childhood Trauma: Historical Casebook and Clinical Applications (#28)
Edited by Jean M. Goodwin, M.D., M.P.H.

Treatment of Adult Survivors of Incest (#27)
Edited by Patricia L. Paddison, M.D.

Madness and Loss of Motherhood: Sexuality, Reproduction, and Long-Term Mental Illness (#26)
Edited by Roberta J. Apfel, M.D., M.P.H., and Maryellen H. Handel, Ph.D.

Psychiatric Aspects of Symptom Management in Cancer Patients (#25)
Edited by William Breitbart, M.D., and Jimmie C. Holland, M.D.

Responding to Disaster: A Guide for Mental Health Professionals (#24)
Edited by Linda S. Austin, M.D.

Psychopharmacological Treatment Complications in the Elderly (#23)
Edited by Charles A. Shamoian, M.D., Ph.D.

Anxiety Disorders in Children and Adolescents (#22)
By Syed Arshad Husain, M.D., F.R.C.P.C., F.R.C.Psych., and Javad Kashani, M.D.

Suicide and Clinical Practice (#21)
Edited by Douglas Jacobs, M.D.

Special Problems in Managing Eating Disorders (#20)
Edited by Joel Yager, M.D., Harry E. Gwirtsman, M.D., and Carole K. Edelstein, M.D.

Children and AIDS (#19)
Edited by Margaret L. Stuber, M.D.

Current Treatments of Obsessive-Compulsive Disorder (#18)
Edited by Michele Tortora Pato, M.D., and Joseph Zohar, M.D.

Benzodiazepines in Clinical Practice: Risks and Benefits (#17)
Edited by Peter P. Roy-Byrne, M.D., and Deborah S. Cowley, M.D.

Adolescent Psychotherapy (#16)
Edited by Marcia Slomowitz, M.D.

Preface

*T*his book is based on a symposium presented at the American Psychiatric Association Annual Conference in San Francisco, California, in May 1993. The symposium was cosponsored with the American Group Psychotherapy Association. Many of the authors in this book have played important roles in both organizations and in the development of group programs across the country. The principal intent of the book is to present a number of models for using therapy groups in a managed care setting.

Randomized clinical trials indicate that the results of group psychotherapy are comparable to those of individual therapy in a broad range of diagnostic categories. The immediate cost effectiveness of groups coupled with this documented positive outcome has made the modality particularly appealing in mental health delivery systems. Unfortunately, there is widespread belief that group therapy is a less powerful, even second-rate, modality that is limited to the provision of general emotional support. This position is not supported by the facts, as I show in Chapter 1 through a review of the available clinical research findings. In this chapter, I also discuss how we can make realistic predictions about the clinical needs that are likely to be encountered when serving a defined clinical population. In Chapter 2, Cross discusses how group therapy can be introduced into managed care settings. Careful attention to this implementation process can make or break the acceptance of group treatments by both clinicians and patients.

There have been many recent developments in research into how group therapy can be most effectively used. In fact, the term *group therapy* carries little specific information about what is actually planned. It is more realistic to consider group therapy as a modality, a vehicle by which a number of different theoretical treatment approaches can be delivered. This book deals with several of these.

In Chapters 3 and 4, Piper and Rice, respectively, deal with time-limited outpatient groups. This format is emerging as a major component in many programs. The combination of a group approach with a definite time limit is appealing from the standpoint of cost containment. However, available outcome data suggest that this combination is also a highly effective way of delivering interpersonal therapies. The program described by Piper has been the subject of sophisticated outcome research, some of which is documented in Chapter 3. In Chapter 4, Rice describes a different kind of time-limited group that is designed to treat a less psychologically sophisticated patient population. It draws in a creative manner on a number of techniques, many from the cognitive-behavioral field. These are packaged together to form a progressively deeper experience for group members.

In Chapters 5 and 6, Peterson and Melson, respectively, describe two models for intensive day treatment programs. These relatively short-term approaches have major advantages in managing patients who might otherwise require inpatient admission. They also incorporate a variety of adjunctive techniques that heighten the intensity level of the psychotherapeutic work. This makes it possible to address quite resistant defenses effectively, a unique advantage of group methods that incorporate a strong emphasis on group process.

Long-term patient populations are dealt with next. In Chapter 7, Stone describes a group-based approach for the seriously mentally ill. Groups offer many advantages over individual therapy for this population. The support and understanding available among the members provides an important sustaining quality. Segal and Weideman, in Chapter 8, describe a unique program for managing patients with severe personality disorders. These patients place a heavy load on service systems. The program described in Chapter 8 provides an effective method for containing and settling such patients over time. It is particularly well suited to the patient with borderline personality disorder features.

In Chapter 9, Kibel puts group therapy into perspective for the future. It is likely that the use of group methods will increase dramatically in organized service settings, providing an opportunity to design effective programs. If such programs are designed improperly, there is the risk of creating situations in which groups conducted by inadequately trained clinicians would become a dumping ground for difficult patients. This would be an injustice both to the patients and to the potential of group methods. It is our hope that this book will provide some useful concepts and models for the practicing clinician and program administrator.

K. Roy MacKenzie, M.D., F.R.C.P.C.

Chapter 1

Rationale for Group Psychotherapy in Managed Care

K. Roy MacKenzie, M.D., F.R.C.P.C.

*T*he delivery of health care services is undergoing serious review throughout the Western world. The increasing costs of advanced technology, coupled with rising public expectations and a time of economic retrenchment, have resulted in fiscal pressures that must be addressed. Different national systems have adopted different strategies for dealing with these issues.

In the United Kingdom, with its National Health Service, there have been vigorous attempts to introduce market strategies. General practitioners now serve as the entry point into the health care system, whereas most specialists are located in hospitals. General practitioners solicit bids from specialists and hospitals for the most economical provision of services for the patients in their practice. There is a safety valve through the existence of a private practice system for those able to afford it, but the government service is itself running into serious limitations in accessibility. This situation clearly suggests the emergence of a two-tiered system of access to health benefits.

In Canada and Germany, universal health insurance systems are also coming under financial review. Because virtually all health services are paid through a single system, various proposals for limiting the range of services or the number of practitioners in a specific area are being considered. In Canada, for example, medical practitioners must work either entirely within the system or entirely outside of it. Some provinces are considering mechanisms to limit the number of practicing physicians billing the health plan. Although access to all is maintained, some areas of specialized services are experiencing growing waiting lists. The virtual absence of private medical resources is increasing pressure on the government system.

The European countries are able to provide general health services at a cost roughly half that of the United States. Canada has historically been ranked as slightly more expensive than Europe. The difference between costs in the United States and those in other Western countries is generally considered to be a result of the entrepreneurial nature of the United States approach, with a higher cost structure related to marketing, administrative functions, and the increased use of high-tech procedures. There is also a greater percentage of specialists in the United States, approximately 70% compared with 50% in other Western countries. This is believed to result in a greater use of expensive investigative procedures.

The inevitable result in all Western countries will undoubtedly be a closer examination of what medical services should be covered. Similarly, there will be an increased focus on how to deliver services in the most economical manner. There may be some consolation in knowing that the problem is not specific to any one country.

The United States is unique among developed countries in not having a comprehensive approach to the organization of health services. This has resulted in a dichotomized system, with services of high excellence existing in parallel with services of questionable quality. It is no surprise that the federal government has health care reform as a high priority. This would undoubtedly be the case no matter which political party was in power, because of social pressure. The task is a much larger and more controversial one than in most other countries because of the highly compartmentalized and competitive nature of the present system. Major changes already in place are transforming the health care landscape. Indeed, the major conceptual shifts are likely to be firmly established in practice well before any federal legislation is passed.

Most health services in the United States are now provided through some sort of managed care structure (Kessler 1989). These structures provide various types of controls on who is covered and how services are utilized. The term *managed care* is a loose one, referring to approaches designed to manage a health care system, as opposed to treating an individual patient. Most Western countries have, in fact, been operating in various forms of "managed care" for some time. The need to control spiraling costs while improving access to health services has given this approach particular urgency in the United States over the last decade. It is helpful to bear in mind that large multi-specialty clinics have been operating in this mode for many years. Now this style of administrative thinking is embracing the entire health care system.

A major shift in orientation is required to put these changes into perspective. The revolution occurring in the United States health care system can be understood as the response to the necessity of providing care for a defined population base. This base can be a corporation, an industry, or a geographic area. Financial pressures have led insurers to be increasingly selective in whom they register, resulting in more people without effective coverage. This has eroded the original insurance principle that risk should be spread evenly across a large population. One response to these developments is an emphasis on ensuring that a defined package of basic benefits is made available to all.

Private-sector health providers are understandably concerned about how to market their resources. Their goal is to maximize the use of available facilities and personnel. This has resulted in the development of services of high excellence that attract patients because of their reputation. The downside has been the emergence of excess capacity in some areas, resulting in expensive marketing strategies, as well as promoting unnecessary use of expensive resources or services. The incentive system promotes the provision of unlimited care based on patient demand and capacity to pay.

Current fiscal pressures focus on the need to balance financial resources with the cost of health care of the defined population. This stands current practice on its head. The issue shifts away from how to attract enough patients to fill the available service capacity to how to reasonably meet the needs of a given population with the available financial resources. This forces a painful review, first of what constitutes necessary medical treatment and second of how such care can be provided most effectively for the betterment of the target population as a whole. Inevitably in this process, there are restrictions of some sort. Goodman et al. (1992) described this succinctly as a "broadening of the healthcare practitioner's duties from private responsibility to public accountability"—a major paradigm shift.

The most widespread restriction of medical resources is currently based on social class. In general, those who can afford insurance coverage have access to a much broader array of services than those who must rely on public-sector programs. Increasingly, even those who have insurance coverage are experiencing the introduction of service limitations based on criteria such as bed utilization or number of office visits. The end result is a greater curtailment of access in the United States than is experienced in most Western countries. Health care is cited as one of the most pressing worries of the general population; it affects hiring practices and decisions about changing jobs and promotes reluctance to use preventive services.

The state of Oregon pioneered public discussion about what should constitute basic health benefits based on effectiveness and life expectancy. In the Oregon plan, medical illnesses are ranked in terms of priority, and those below a cutoff point are not eligible for reimbursement; most psychiatric conditions are above that point. Discussions about topics such as those raised in the Oregon plan are preoccupying all levels of the private and public health industry, though not usually in as open a fashion.

The mental health component of the general health system is no exception to all of these trends in health care. Indeed, it is at greater risk than many other specialty areas. Historically, mental health care has been separated from the mainstream of medicine. Today there are some who argue that there is a difference between biological psychiatry and psychological psychiatry and that only the former should qualify as an insurable benefit. This is a serious threat to the "talking" treatments.

Clinical Research Issues

Research funding has been overwhelmingly in the area of psychopharmacology. Unidimensional outcome measures with a narrow focus on specific symptoms have been the general rule, with little or no attention paid to overall adaptation (e.g., the measurement of depression with only the patient's report based on the Beck Depression Inventory). Very short follow-up time periods (e.g., 4–6 weeks) are common. In contrast, the current psychotherapy research literature has emphasized the importance of a multidimensional outcome battery that includes the perspectives of the patient, the therapist, and an independent assessor, and it is increasingly expected that measures of general social/vocational functioning be included as well.

Relatively few studies have attempted to compare psychosocial to pharmacological treatments. In those that have, surprisingly contradictory results have emerged. There is a general trend showing that the more stringent the treatment protocol, the less difference there is between therapies (Elkin et al. 1988a, 1988b). This includes such technical considerations as effective blinding in the use of a control group, a form of active treatment for the control patients, the use of independent assessments of change, and a longer follow-up period. When these requirements are met, different treatments appear to have relatively similar outcomes, indicating a large common effect.

One of the largest and most comprehensive studies of comparative treatments was the National Institute of Mental Health's (NIMH) Collaborative Study of Depression (Elkin et al. 1989). Patients with major depression were randomized into four treatment conditions: administration of imipramine, interpersonal psychotherapy, cognitive-behavior therapy, and placebo and clinical management. The latter condition consisted of active control treatment that included weekly 15- to 20-minute visits. All treatments lasted 16 weeks. The patients' depression responded well to all four treatment approaches. Only when severity within the major depressive range was factored into the analysis were there major differential treatment effects. The most severely ill patients in the imipramine and interpersonal psychotherapy groups showed a significant positive response. The cognitive-behavior therapy group was only a bit behind. The severely ill patients in the control group did significantly less well.

The study of psychotherapy is hampered by an inadequate set of diagnostic criteria. The artificial division between Axis I syndrome categories and Axis II personality disorders obscures the clinical impression that there are major therapeutically relevant connections between them. For example, dysthymia on Axis I has many features of long-standing personality disorder on Axis II. The introduction of Axis II as a formal part of the diagnostic system has been a mixed blessing. On the one hand, it has brought a renewed interest in the study of personality disorders. On the other hand, the nature of the current Axis II category system is not supported by empirical data (Livesley and Jackson 1992). Numerous studies have demonstrated a large overlap between categories of personality disorder (Loranger et al. 1987; Pfohl et al. 1986). This overlap occurs in part because a number of the descriptive criteria are common to more than one diagnostic category; for example, an acute sensitivity to loss of a relationship is found in both borderline personality disorder and dependent personality disorder (Morey 1988).

A dimensional system of character traits would be more in accord with research findings (Wiggins and Trapnell 1992). For example, many anxiety disorders are superimposed on a character style that is highly loaded on a neuroticism dimension. This is a well-defined character pattern that appears nowhere in the formal nomenclature. The use of a dimensional diagnostic system, coupled with a solid measure of functional performance similar to Axis V, appears to be an emerging solution. This would make it more practical to design treatment programs that target particular goals. These theoretical problems are particularly relevant to the use of group psychotherapy because it is especially well suited to the treatment of dysfunctional character pathology.

The pressures for cost containment, together with more sophisticated psychotherapy outcome studies, put into focus several key questions regarding the provision of mental health care. What is the necessity for a particular treatment? What is its effectiveness? How can this treatment be most efficiently delivered? Psychotherapeutic activities form a substantial component of mental health care. In the following section, I present approaches for considering these questions.

The Psychotherapy Delivery System

The idea of psychotherapy as a treatment within a service delivery system goes against the grain for many psychotherapists. Because psychotherapy involves such a close and personalized relationship with the patient, the thought of regarding it as a service with possible limitations is difficult to accept. In the beginning, psychotherapy was considered a relatively brief process. Freud reported many cases of therapy that lasted fewer than a dozen sessions (Strupp and Binder 1984). With time, the analytic community began to focus more on the interpretation of intrapsychic conflict and the working through of transference, with a decreased focus on the relief of specific symptoms. During the 1950s, the tradition of lengthy and essentially time-unlimited psychotherapy became the norm. The process became more important than the outcome (Marmor 1979).

The pioneering work of practitioners such as Alexander and

French (1946), Balint et al. (1972), Sifneos (1977), Malan (1979), Davanloo (1980), and Mann and Goldman (1987) provided a basis for short-term psychotherapy. These authors stressed the importance of carefully selecting patients for time-limited psychotherapy. For example, Sifneos requires "psychological sophistication," a combination of psychological mindedness and above-average intelligence; by implication, many patients would not qualify.

During the 1980s a trend began of using time-limited psychotherapy as the central treatment modality (Budman and Gurman 1988; MacKenzie 1988). A major review article by Marmor (1979) is the best marker of this shift in emphasis. This was reinforced by published material about how patients actually use psychotherapeutic services and how they respond to treatment. Several meta-analytic studies indicated that the overall response rate to psychotherapy is in the range of an "effect size" of approximately 0.85 Standard Units (Shapiro and Shapiro 1982; Smith et al. 1980). This means that the average treated patient does significantly better than 80% of untreated control subjects (Garfield and Bergin 1986). This response rate is in the same range as that achieved in most medication studies of depression and is based on longer follow-up assessments than those in most psychopharmacology studies.

The time course of improvement is of particular interest. Figure 1–1 is a composite graph that summarizes an extensive data base of nonpsychotic patients attending mental health centers or general hospital outpatient departments. Utilization data (Knesper et al. 1985) indicate that 46% of patients being seen by mental health service providers fall into the diagnostic categories of dysthymia, anxiety, or personality disorder. Another 23% are in the category of major mood disorders and might benefit from a psychotherapeutic component in their treatment. The term *dose-effect curve* was used by Howard et al. (1986) as a deliberate parallel to the pharmacotherapy literature: time in therapy equals dosage. Figure 1–1 can be used as a general map of the psychotherapy utilization terrain. The results of most studies, including the NIMH study cited above, fall into the patterns represented in Figure 1–1.

The top curve in Figure 1–1 is a measure of improvement as determined by objective assessment (Howard et al. 1986). It is thus a conservative measure because patient or therapist ratings are usually more positive than those made by an uninvolved clinician. The curve shows a rapid improvement over the first 2 months, followed by continuing strong improvement over the next 4 months. After that, the curve rises much more slowly for the remaining time up to 2 years. The final response rate is about 85%, quite in keeping with the meta-analytic figures mentioned previously. It might be noted that even patients who are still in treatment 1–2 years later report an early symptomatic response as reflected in the top curve.

The bottom curve in Figure 1–1 is based on a different, but equally large, data base of actual number of sessions attended in a similar patient population (Phillips 1987). The great majority of patients (over 80%) were seen for fewer than eight sessions. Less than 15% were still in treatment at 6 months. After that, there was a strong likelihood that attendance continued over many months more. This curve appears to be quite constant across many different service systems. The exact point of the sharp bend at eight sessions can vary a little, but the rapid initial falloff is universal.

Two more-detailed reports confirm this, both conducted in outpatient clinics where the major theoretical orientation was toward long-term, analytically oriented treatment. In the early days of psychotherapy expansion, Garfield and Kurz (1952) reviewed the case files of 560 patients in such a clinic. They found that two-thirds of the patients attended fewer than 10 sessions, and only 13% remained for more than 20 sessions. More recently, Sledge et al. (1990) reported on a cohort of 69 patients entering long-term therapy. The mean number of sessions actually attended was 15.4. In fact, this represented about one-third who attended for a lengthy time and two-thirds who received quite short-term therapy. In the same study, the authors reported that the dropout rate was much less when a definite time limit was established at the beginning of therapy rather than leaving the termination date vague.

Three distinct phases can be seen in the three sections of Figure 1–1. They correspond quite closely to the major outlines of clinical practice.

1. Crisis Intervention

Crisis intervention occupies the phase up to eight sessions, or approximately 2 months. During this phase, the task is to achieve immediate mastery by focusing on specific, but limited, goals related to promoting a return to usual functioning. Interpersonal or psychodynamic goals can be addressed, but in a focused and more directive manner. As shown in Figure 1–1, it can be quite reliably predicted that about one-half of the unscreened population presenting to psychiatric outpatient settings will derive benefit from this brief therapy, and an even larger percentage will have terminated by the eighth session.

This rapid response is probably related to the fact that patients do not present for care solely because they are symptomatic. Community surveys indicate that many people with diagnosable psychiatric conditions do not seek treatment. Shapiro et al. (1984) found in the Epidemiologic Catchment Area study that only 18% of those diagnosed as having affective disorder and only 11% of those diagnosed as having anxiety or somatoform disorders (according to DSM-III criteria [Amer-

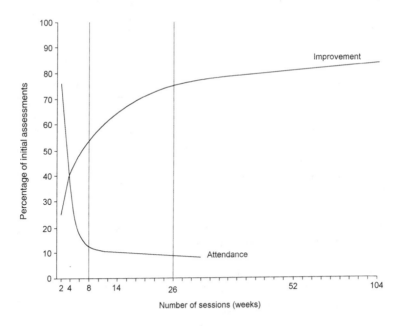

Figure 1–1.   Psychotherapy dose-effect curve.

Source.   Adapted from MacKenzie KR: *Introduction to Time-Limited Group Psychotherapy.* Washington, DC, American Psychiatric Press, 1990, p. 228. Used with permission.

ican Psychiatric Association 1980]) had seen a mental health specialist in the previous 6 months. Instead, people came for help when they reached a point of feeling overwhelmed, often influenced by a sense of hopelessness or demoralization. Many of those patients reacted to stressful events that incorporated a component of loss.

This demoralized state of mind can be rapidly reversed for many people with a small number of psychotherapy sessions. Because a sizable percentage can be expected to respond quickly and because the falloff in attendance is so steep, it has been the custom to use individual therapy in this phase of treatment. Some innovative programs have been applying group techniques during this phase as well.

2. Time-Limited Therapy

The next challenge is to address the needs of the other half of presenting patients who are likely to benefit from a longer treatment course. The second time phase in Figure 1–1 is between 8 and about 25 sessions, or around 6 months. This phase continues to be a time of continuing major improvement. This is the phase that is covered within the usual theoretical framework of time-limited therapy. Several of the examples in this book include this phase. The increased time allows accommodation of higher levels of distress and adjustment to more severe trauma or stress. It can also be used to treat patients whose presentation involves a greater contribution of long-standing issues of a psychological nature. In short, more ambitious goals can be entertained.

In this phase, it would be reasonable to consider programs of at least two types: one that incorporates a fair degree of structure and specific focus and another that uses less-structured interactional or psychodynamically oriented techniques. In either case, a specific deadline is incorporated. A group modality is well suited to this phase. It can be confidently predicted that a sizable additional improvement rate will result (Piper et al. 1992).

3. Longer-Term Therapy

Beyond 6 months we move into the range of longer-term treatment. Patients who are still in therapy at this point tend to continue for many more months or years. Improvement continues but the pace of change becomes slower. The balance between active change and maintenance functions begins to shift toward the latter. Here, again, one can describe

two types of groups. Some are designed for long-term, "eternal" maintenance functions in which major change is not likely, but support and
containment are quite helpful. The goal is to prevent decompensation
and hospitalization. An example would be a community program for
more severely schizophrenic individuals. Other long-term programs are
designed for ongoing active treatment of more severe problems, such
as major personality disorders, but for which eventual discharge is
anticipated. Even in this category, the containing effects of ongoing
treatment can result in a considerable cost benefit because of a reduction in use of emergency room and inpatient bed resources.

The above categorization of treatment phases does not, of course,
apply to every individual patient. However, it is a quite reliable description of how service systems operate (Howard et al. 1992). It can be used
to predict the sort of resources that are likely to be required for a
specific population base. Programs for specific diagnostic populations
might have different characteristics, but it is interesting how closely
most programs approximate the utilization patterns shown in Figure
1–1. Therapists tend to remember those patients they have seen for a
substantial length of time. Those who pass through quickly are just as
quickly forgotten. From the patient's standpoint, however, even a brief
encounter of a few sessions is sometimes described as a point of
significant change in how they approach life's challenges.

Using the three-phase model above, it is possible to identify specific critical decision points. At the time of initial assessment, a preliminary decision is required about the probable nature of the time contact
needed. A second decision point occurs at the end of a few sessions
(e.g., six or eight). A third and more serious decision point is appropriate after a longer period (e.g., between 4 and 6 months). It is helpful
when looking at a service delivery system to incorporate these sequen-
tial decisions into standard operating procedures. Even for the solo
practitioner, it can be useful to think of treatment expectations in terms
of these time categories.

Some patients with a history of satisfactory premorbid functioning
and the presence of an acute stressor can be channeled immediately into
a crisis intervention mode with a clearly specified time limit. Others
might be considered for a formal time-limited contract of several
months to work on specific issues. A common decision might be to see
the patient for a few sessions to test capacity and motivation. If more
time is required, these sessions provide useful preparation for more

intensive, but time-limited, treatment. The principal danger is that if the original therapist is not going to provide the next treatment phase, the transition can be difficult for the patient, with a substantial likelihood of unplanned termination. Similarly, if group treatment is recommended, the transition from individual treatment can be viewed quite negatively. The earlier the decision is made and discussed with the patient, the less likely it is that transition problems will occur.

Other patients can be channeled immediately at initial evaluation into the long-term treatment stream because of past history and diagnostic category. To put such patients into a brief program would be of little therapeutic value to them and indeed would be a waste of clinical resources. Patients with a major mental illness such as schizophrenia or bipolar disorder need treatment planning that is long-term in nature. Patients exhibiting a major personality disorder accompanied by significant dysfunction in many areas are also unlikely to respond to briefer modalities. Unfortunately, the current Axis II diagnostic criteria are of limited value in making these decisions (Livesley and Jackson 1992). The clinician is better advised to consider other dimensions.

The level of chaos or destructiveness in close relationships can reflect enduring severe personality pathology. The ability to maintain employment and to function as a reasonably active person in the community with a nucleus of friends is reflected in the Global Assessment of Functioning Scale (Axis V of DSM-III-R [American Psychiatric Association 1987]). Low ratings on such criteria identify a long-standing and pervasive level of dysfunction. There is currently some enthusiasm for treating characterological difficulties using time-limited approaches if the present state reflects a decompensation from usual levels of coping, even if such a decompensation has occurred before. Axis IV ratings of objective psychosocial stressors are useful for this assessment.

Groups in the Mental Health System

This book is focused on one aspect of the managed health care system: the way in which group therapy can be most effectively utilized. Clearly, the use of a group format offers immediate cost efficiency. However, serious questions must be answered. Are groups as effective as individual approaches? How much time needs to be spent in a group for effective results? What sorts of patients are suited for what sorts of groups? Can groups be successfully incorporated as a routine component in service settings? Will patient resistance limit the use of groups? Can clinicians adapt to the additional clinical skills required for effective management of a group?

Historically, the use of group therapy methods has waxed and waned (Scheidlinger and Schamess 1992). Before World War II, the systematic use of groups was rare. The need to treat large numbers of service personnel experiencing stress reactions led to the widespread development of group therapy methods. Not coincidentally, the American Group Psychotherapy Association (AGPA) was formed in 1942. W. C. Menninger, America's Chief of Military Psychiatry, felt that the development of group therapy was one of the major contributions of military psychiatry to civilian practice (Menninger 1946).

The 1960s and 1970s saw another surge of interest in the use of group therapy. This was in part related to the passage of the Community Mental Health Center (CMHC) Act in 1963 with its promise of a "Third Mental Health Revolution." The intent was to develop a mental health service system open to all. The enthusiasm for the development of CMHCs gradually faded. Some CMHCs focused primarily on acute problems, whereas the more difficult problems of patients at lower socioeconomic levels and chronic patients, primarily with schizophrenia, were again left to the side. Other CMHCs experienced controversy over the use of less-qualified clinicians running groups that became either less effective or more troublesome. These developments ran in parallel with the unprecedented explosion of group-based modalities in the community under the headings of "encounter groups" or "T-groups." This blurring of approaches between the reasonably well-functioning population and those with identified dysfunctional illness resulted in a general discrediting of group therapy. Groups were seen as having little specific value in terms of formal treatment expectations. Indeed, the use of group therapy in clinical settings began to decline. This decline was augmented by the major swing of organized psychiatry into biological models of etiology and treatment.

The role of groups in mental treatment is again increasing in prominence. This trend has been fueled both by controlled research studies on effectiveness and by economic considerations. We are entering the third age of group therapy: Whereas the first age was driven by wartime necessity and the second age was created by a general social swing toward experiential events, this third and current age is the result of more sober considerations of a scientific and economic nature. As a reflection of this swing, attendance at group-related presentations at national meetings has increased, group organizations such as AGPA are experiencing an expansion of membership, and the number of books and journal articles devoted to group therapy topics has expanded.

Comparing Individual and Group Therapy

Group therapy techniques have historically been seen as a secondary treatment modality, certainly not on the same level as the "gold standard" of individual therapy. This opinion tends to be shared by patients. Most practitioners are surprised to learn that there is substantial literature comparing the two approaches. In the first major meta-analytic study of psychotherapy effectiveness (Smith et al. 1980), approximately half of the 475 studies were taken from the group therapy literature. The outcome results for group therapy are basically similar to the upper improvement line in Figure 1–1. In a recent study, Piper et al. (1992), using a waiting list control design, found highly significant treatment effects. This study is of particular interest because the groups were quite brief (12 sessions) but run with an intensive psychodynamic approach.

Toseland and Siporin (1986) reviewed 32 studies that met rigorous criteria for research design. In these studies, patients were randomized into group or individual therapy treatment using the same theoretical approach. In 75% of the studies (24 of the 32), there was no statistical difference in outcome between group and individual therapy. In the remaining 8 studies, group therapy was found to be more effective. In no case was group treatment found to be less effective than individual therapy. Orlinsky and Howard (1986) reported on 14 comparisons between group and individual approaches; in 11 there was no difference. In 3 of the comparisons, individual therapy was more effective, but 2 of these situations were with inpatient schizophrenic patients—not an ideal group for psychotherapeutic treatment.

More recently, Tillitski (1990) has reported a meta-analysis from nine studies with a total of 349 subjects that contrasted group, individual, and control treatments in a pre- and posttest design. The "effect sizes" were even larger than those found by Smith et al. (1980). Both group and individual therapy effects were about twice as large as those for controls. There was little difference between the two modalities, although group therapy seemed more effective with adolescents and individual treatment more effective with children. Several other controlled studies have specifically compared group with individual treatment and found no difference on pre- and posttest measures (Budman et al. 1988; Pilkonis et al. 1984; Piper et al. 1984).

At the very least, these results suggest that group therapy is clearly not a second-rate treatment. These effectiveness data, combined with the relative efficiency of the group therapy modality, make a powerful argument for more extensive use of groups in service delivery settings. In one of the studies cited above (Piper et al. 1984), patients were randomly assigned to four treatment approaches: brief (24 sessions over 6 months) and long-term (96 sessions over 2 years) treatment with individual or group therapy. All four formats used a psychodynamic orientation and all achieved very positive outcome results. A calculation was made of the relative efficiency of the four treatments. The therapist time ratios per patient for the four conditions were as follows: short-term group = 1; long-term group = 4; short-term individual = 5; long-term individual = 20.

The term *group therapy* does not in itself carry great meaning. Groups can be more accurately seen as a modality for delivering a variety of theoretical material. Much of the group therapy literature has been devoted to relatively unstructured interpersonal or psychodynamic methods. However, increasing numbers of reports are available regarding the use of groups to provide cognitive-behavior therapy (Linehan 1993). Groups have for many years been the primary method for presenting psychoeducational material (Davis et al. 1992). Groups can also be used to deliver the semistructured type of interpersonal therapy used in the NIMH depression study (Klerman et al. 1984). In all of these applications, proper attention to the management of the group environment can enhance the effectiveness the particular approach being used.

Groups bring with them some powerful basic therapeutic mechanisms that serve in their own right to increase morale and motivate patients (Yalom 1985). The sense of universality that is found early in a group combats feelings of isolation and strangeness. The experience of being accepted in a group despite one's experiences, symptoms, and behaviors is an antidote to demoralization. Groups also provide an opportunity to help others and this experience of altruism enhances self-esteem. All of these factors work together to help develop a sense of greater mastery over self and problems. Specific technical aspects of the treatment can use these common group factors to augment the nature of the treatment. This phenomenon is parallel to the importance of the "therapeutic alliance" in individual therapy. The nature of the "group alliance" is more complex and multifaceted. It is less focused on the therapist and thus less likely to create undue dependence on authority. No matter what their purpose, all groups have at their disposal these therapeutic qualities. Because of the identification of group therapy with psychodynamic theories, therapists of other theoretical persuasions are sometimes reluctant to acknowledge these properties of the group. Even though they can describe them as present and interesting, they may be unsure about how to maximize their potential.

Designing Treatment Programs

The information given above is of value when considering how a managed care treatment program might be structured in terms of the "talking" component. Group therapy is particularly well suited to larger service systems. A setting in which several practitioners can refer patients to groups provides access to a larger flow of patients. Thus, groups can be designed for special purposes without always having to wait until enough potential members can be accumulated. For example, a system might want to have a constant accessibility to general time-limited interpersonal groups that can serve a broad segment of the nonpsychotic population. With a large enough referral base, such groups could be planned to start every month or two, depending on the predictable numbers of referrals. Thus, referring clinicians would be able to book patients into a group after only a relatively brief waiting period. Similarly, special groups for cognitive-behavioral treatment of depressed patients could be organized, or groups for psychoeducational services for patients with eating disorders. A long-term group for containing difficult patients in the community with the goal of achieving a lower rate of acute admissions might be considered. Each system would need to analyze its own needs and conceptualize how many groups would probably be required in the course of a year. With this sort of preplanning, the use of the available group therapists can be maximized.

The vertical lines shown in Figure 1–1 have been used to suggest ways of segmenting the time dimension of therapy. Three time categories are indicated: crisis intervention with firm limits on the number of individual sessions, time-limited groups, and long-term groups. These statistically derived time segments appear to be quite robust across different clinical settings. They do not, of course, predict which individual patient is going to fall into which time category, but they do provide a reasonable method for predicting the probable distribution of service resources.

These patterns can be applied to the utilization of staff time. Table 1–1 illustrates how staff time is distributed depending on whether individual or group modalities were used to deliver therapy in the last two time segments. Calculations are based on the maximum time figures in each time segment, which is probably an overly generous figure. The first four columns indicate how the utilization picture looks when only individual therapy is used. More than one-third of the available clinical time is spent on the 15% of long-term patients. The last two columns show the change when group therapy is used to treat

Table 1–1.   Hypothetical utilization of staff time comparing individual versus group modalities for 100 patients

Patients in each time segment (%)[a]	Mean number of sessions per time segment[a]	Individual therapy		Group therapy	
		Total hours per 100 patients	% of staff resources	Total hours per 100 patients	% of staff resources
50	8	400	20	400 (unchanged)	50
35	25	875	43	200 (4 groups)	25
15	50	750	37	200 (2 groups)	25
100	—	2,025	100	800	100

[a]See Figure 1–1.

those in the time-limited and long-term categories. It is assumed that all groups are solo led and that each 90-minute group occupies 2 hours of clinician time. The overall clinician time utilization drops to 40%. The percentage of staff time devoted to the 50% acute, but brief, contact patients more than doubles. Even allowing for rather generous time limits, the mean number of sessions for all patients is 8 visits when group methods are used for the more time-intensive portion of treatment, compared with a mean of 20 visits when only individual therapy is used. These numbers need not be taken at exactly face value because there will be many justifiable exceptions, but they do show the potential magnitude of change involved.

The principles outlined above regarding the time components of psychotherapy can be built into organizational structures. For example, by putting a limit on the number of individual crisis-oriented sessions, a specialized service component can be designed for this purpose, with a clear mandate to keep a very specific focus and the goal of reestablishing stability, not major psychological change. A specific decision can then be made to shift the patient into a more intensive but time-limited program. This is a format to which groups are well suited. Perhaps the most critical decision of all is to determine which patients require long-term treatment. This is where the cost in terms of clinical resources increases significantly. It would be the point at which some sort of formal review process might be introduced. Long-term referrals can be predicted to be appropriate for about 15% of original patients in most systems. This program component would be especially important for patients who are high users of health care resources. If inpatient care and use of emergency services can be reduced, the financial cost of long-term group therapy is well justified. Studies have suggested that adequate psychiatric treatment can result in a substantial reduction in general medical costs (Budman et al. 1988; Mumford et al. 1984).

Patients are likely to be skeptical about a referral for group therapy. Their principal exposure to groups might well have been through media presentations where humor or sensationalism was the dominant force. The first mention made of the possibility of group treatment is a critical point. A positive and constructive attitude must be demonstrated. Any comment suggesting even slightly that groups are being recommended because of cost pressures will elicit a predictable sense of outrage. That is why the scientific information about group effectiveness has been discussed in some detail earlier in this chapter. It well behooves the clinician to be able to review this material knowledgeably, not in exact numbers, but in terms of its overall message. This clinical discussion with the patient about group treatment can also make reference to the learned nature of many interpersonal patterns and attitudes about self.

Groups offer a more powerful and complex interpersonal environment than dyadic therapy. A handout written in lay language about the myths associated with group therapy and the beneficial effects of groups can be given to the patient for reading and subsequent discussion (for a sample, see MacKenzie 1990). The clinician should anticipate that the patient will have concerns, and these must be non-defensively elicited. Most concerns are quite predictable: that groups are a second-rate treatment; that members will be forced to make confessions; that they will get worse because of emotional contagion from other members; that the group will get out of control; or that one will be rejected by the other members as being too sick or too unusual for them to understand. In fact, most of these statements are the exact opposite of what is likely to happen. When a program finds it is having difficulty persuading patients to accept a group approach, the problem almost always resides in the attitude of the staff or the lack of systematic pretherapy preparation procedures.

Most of the clinical programs described in this book entail a brief format. As such, they share in the general tradition of time-limited psychotherapy. The essential components of all of these techniques can be summarized in a few basic principles:

1. Careful assessment should determine the patient's capacity to use the format being utilized.
2. An explicit agreement regarding circumscribed goals should be negotiated openly with the patient before treatment begins.
3. The therapist should intervene actively to develop a therapeutic group climate.
4. The therapist should be active in maintaining a working focus on the goals identified.
5. The establishment of a time limit will increase the tempo of work.
6. The therapist should encourage application of the learning to the present, both within the group and in current outside circumstances.

7. The therapist should encourage and expect patient responsibility for initiating therapy tasks.
8. The process of termination and dealing with the time limit needs to be a major focus during the last half of the group.
9. It is anticipated that change will continue after termination of therapy, so all problematic issues do not need to be addressed within the therapeutic context.

Developing Group Skills

Some therapists who have been primarily trained in individual therapy can make the transition to the group situation smoothly. However, most experience some difficulty. The most common error is to move without conscious effort into treating individual patients in a group context. This may not be actively harmful, although it can demoralize the group and lead to premature dropouts. At the very least, such an error fails to capitalize on the energy of the group to promote the therapeutic factors mentioned earlier in this chapter. This results in less-effective treatment. Group therapy, like individual therapy, can be harmful. This usually involves mishandling of affectively laden material. For example, disclosure of powerful personal material that receives no validation or response can be quite devastating. Anger, particularly anger in which the therapist directly or indirectly colludes, can create a scapegoating pattern that is particularly damaging. Issues surrounding subgrouping between members can also be hazardous. In short, group management skills are important when treating a group population that is by definition experiencing psychological difficulties.

The basic components of group management are often not adequately presented or supervised in professional training programs. Clinicians need to receive a basic introduction to the theory of small groups. Such an introduction helps to make the transition from individual to group treatment smoother and equips the clinician to identify group-level phenomena. Personal experience in an experiential training group is highly recommended as a powerful way to become more attuned to the nuances of group dynamics.

The most important training component is to receive regular, detailed supervision while running a group. Such supervision can be accomplished in various ways. Participating as a cotherapist with an experienced group clinician provides an opportunity to become more comfortable in the group environment and to model therapy skills. Although some care needs to be taken in regard to perceived role imbalance, this is usually not a serious problem if there is a good working understanding between the two therapists. Supervision provided by direct observation is another common method; many of the same advantages can be found using videotaped sessions. Common to all of these approaches is the use of actual observation of the group process. This is most important. The group arena is more complex than individual therapy and it is possible for quite major group dynamics to be missed by the neophyte group therapist. This is possible, perhaps even more likely, when the therapist has a background in individual psychotherapy. There can be no substitute for the direct observation of groups by the clinical supervisor.

The most important new clinical learning in the transition from individual therapy usually centers around being able to conceptualize the group as a whole in addition to understanding the individual patients. Only with this accomplished can the therapist knowledgeably choose between intrapsychic, interpersonal, or group-level interventions. Group therapy training opportunities are found in many major cities. They can also be obtained through professional meetings, such as those sponsored by the AGPA and its affiliated societies.

In addition to proper training, it is important for clinicians running groups to have an opportunity to discuss their work with colleagues. The group environment can exert quite powerful pressures on the leader, and it is easy to temporarily get pulled off of a therapeutic position of neutrality. The chance to talk about situations and personal reactions is usually adequate to provide a stabilizing correction. It is best if peer consultation is not something that is sought only in emergencies. Most group difficulties arise over time and can be forestalled at an early point if detected and discussed. One approach that is both effective and efficient is a regular clinical seminar conducted by an experienced group therapist. If an atmosphere of trust and openness is created, such a seminar can meet the needs of a sizable number of staff. Many programs use a 1-hour weekly time slot for this function. It must be given support and time priority by the program director. Encouragement might also be given for involvement in local and national group therapy organizations in which a broader exposure to aspects of clinical practice can be found.

Summary

In this chapter, I have emphasized the importance of conceptualizing service delivery systems, rather than the individual patient. Group therapy is a demonstrably effective treatment modality. The larger flow of patients within treatment systems allows the design of group-based programs in accordance with the clinical needs of the population being served. Well-established service patterns can be used to estimate these needs. The increase in efficiency provided by groups, together with their proven effectiveness, provides a powerful argument for their use. Indeed, it would be reasonable to suggest that group therapy should form the primary modality for planned time-limited psychotherapy following a brief crisis-intervention phase. Groups are particularly helpful for that small proportion of patients who require long-term management to decrease utilization in other aspects of the system. Given the comparability of outcomes, health benefit guidelines should be adjusted to allow for a higher ratio of group to individual sessions. Alternatively, a lower copayment for group therapy would provide incentive for maximizing the greater efficiency of the group modality.

References

Alexander F, French TM: Psychoanalytic Therapy: Principles and Application (1946). Lincoln, NE, University of Nebraska Press, 1980

American Psychiatric Association: Diagnostic and Statistical Manual of Mental Disorders, 3rd Edition. Washington, DC, American Psychiatric Association, 1980

Balint M, Ornstein PH, Balint E: Focal Psychotherapy. London, Tavistock, 1972

Budman SH, Demby A, Redondo JP, et al: Comparative outcome in time-limited individual and group psychotherapy. Int J Group Psychother 38:63–86, 1988

Budman SH, Gurman AS: Theory and Practice of Brief Therapy. New York, Guilford, 1988

Davanloo H (ed): Short-Term Dynamic Psychotherapy. New York, Aronson, 1980

Davis R, Dearing S, Faulkner J, et al: The road to recovery: a manual for participants in the psychoeducational group for bulimia nervosa, in Group Psychotherapy for Eating Disorders. Edited by Harper-Giuffre H, MacKenzie KR. Washington, DC, American Psychiatric Press, 1992, pp 271–342

Elkin I, Pilkonis PA, Docherty JP, et al: Conceptual and methodological issues in comparative studies of psychotherapy and pharmacotherapy, I: active ingredients and mechanisms of change. Am J Psychiatry 145:909–917, 1988a

Elkin I, Pilkonis PA, Docherty JP, et al: Conceptual and methodological issues in comparative studies of psychotherapy and pharmacotherapy, II: nature and timing of treatment effects. Am J Psychiatry 145:1070–1076, 1988b

Elkin I, Shea MT, Watkins JT, et al: National Institute of Mental Health treatment of depression collaborative research program: general effectiveness of treatments. Arch Gen Psychiatry 46:971–982, 1989

Garfield SL, Bergin AE (eds): Handbook of Psychotherapy and Behavior Change. New York, Wiley, 1986

Garfield SL, Kurz M: Evaluation of treatment and related procedures in 1,216 cases referred to a mental hygiene clinic. Psychiatr Q 26:412–424, 1952

Goodman M, Brown J, Deitz P: Managing Managed Care: A Mental Health Practitioner's Survival Guide. Washington, DC, American Psychiatric Press, 1992

Howard KI, Kopta SM, Krause MS, et al: The dose-effect relationship in psychotherapy. Am Psychol 41:159–164, 1986

Howard KI, Lueger R, Schank D: The psychotherapeutic service delivery system. Psychotherapy Research 2:164–180, 1992

Kessler K: Managed psychiatric care will continue to boom. Clinical Psychiatry News 17:6–7, 1989

Klerman GL, Weissman MM, Rounsaville BJ, et al: Interpersonal Psychotherapy of Depression. New York, Basic Books, 1984

Knesper DJ, Pagnucco DJ, Wheeler JR: Similarities and differences across mental health services providers and practice settings in the United States. Am Psychol 40:1352–1369, 1985

Linehan MM: Cognitive-Behavioral Treatment of Borderline Personality Disorder. New York, Guilford, 1993

Livesley WJ, Jackson DN: Guidelines for developing, evaluating, and revising the classification of personality disorders. J Nerv Ment Dis 180:609–618, 1992

Loranger AW, Susman VL, Oldham JM, et al: The personality disorder examination. Journal of Personality Disorders 1:1–13, 1987

MacKenzie KR: Recent developments in brief psychotherapy. Hosp Community Psychiatry 39:742–752, 1988

MacKenzie KR: Introduction to Time-Limited Group Psychotherapy. Washington, DC, American Psychiatric Press, 1990

Malan DH: Individual Psychotherapy and the Science of Psychodynamics, 2nd Edition. London, Butterworth, 1979

Mann J, Goldman R: A Casebook in Time-Limited Psychotherapy (1982). Washington, DC, American Psychiatric Press, 1987

Marmor J: Short-term dynamic psychotherapy. Am J Psychiatry 136:149–155, 1979

Menninger WC: Lessons from military psychiatry for civilian psychiatry. Mental Hygiene 30:571–580, 1946

Morey LC: Personality disorders in DSM-III and DSM-III-R: Convergence, coverage, and internal consistency. Am J Psychiatry 145:573–577, 1988

Mumford E, Schlesinger HJ, Glass GV, et al: A new look at evidence about reduced cost of medical utilization following mental health treatment. Am J Psychiatry 141:1145–1158, 1984

Orlinsky DE, Howard KI: Process and outcome in psychotherapy, in Handbook of Psychotherapy and Behavior Change, 3rd Edition. Edited by Garfield SL, Bergin AE. New York, Wiley, 1986, pp 311–381

Pfohl B, Coryell W, Zimmerman M, et al: DSM-III personality disorders: diagnostic overlap and internal consistency of individual DSM-III criteria. Compr Psychiatry 27:21–34, 1986

Phillips EL: The ubiquitous decay curve: delivery similarities in psychotherapy, medicine and addiction. Professional Psychology: Research and Practice 18:650–652, 1987

Pilkonis PA, Imber SD, Lewis P, et al: A comparative outcome study of individual, group, and conjoint psychotherapy. Arch Gen Psychiatry 41:431–437, 1984

Piper WE, Debbane EG, Bienvenu JP, et al: A comparative study of four forms of psychotherapy. J Consult Clin Psychol 52:268–279, 1984

Piper WE, McCallum M, Azim HFA: Adaptation to Loss Through Short-Term Group Therapy. New York, Guilford, 1992

Scheidlinger S, Schamess G: Fifty years of AGPA 1942–1992: an overview, in Classics in Group Psychotherapy. Edited by MacKenzie KR. New York, Guilford, 1992, pp 1–22

Shapiro DA, Shapiro D: Meta-analysis of comparative therapy outcome studies: a replication and refinement. Psychol Bull 92:581–604, 1982

Shapiro S, Skinner EA, Kessler LG, et al: Utilization of health and mental health services: three Epidemiologic Catchment Area sites. Arch Gen Psychiatry 41:971–978, 1984

Sifneos PE: Short-Term Dynamic Psychotherapy, 2nd Edition. New York, Plenum, 1987

Sledge WH, Moras K, Hartley D, et al: Effect of time-limited psychotherapy on patient dropout rates. Am J Psychiatry 147:1341–1347, 1990

Smith ML, Glass GV, Miller TI: The Benefits of Psychotherapy. Baltimore, MD, Johns Hopkins University Press, 1980

Strupp HH, Binder JL: Psychotherapy in a New Key: A Guide to Time-Limited Dynamic Psychotherapy. New York, Basic Books, 1984

Tillitski CJ: A meta-analysis of estimated effect size for group vs. individual vs. control treatments. Int J Group Psychother 40:215–224, 1990

Toseland RW, Siporin M: When to recommend group treatment: a review of the clinical and the research literature. Int J Group Psychother 36:171–201, 1986

Weiner MF: Group therapy reduces medical and psychiatric hospitalization. Int J Group Psychother 42:267–275, 1992

Wiggins JS, Trapnell PD: Personality structure: the return of the Big Five, in Handbook of Personality Pathology. Edited by Briggs MS, Hogan R, Jones W. Orlando FL, Academic Press, 1992

Yalom ID: The Theory and Practice of Group Psychotherapy, 3rd Edition. New York, Basic Books, 1985

Chapter 2

Organizing Group Psychotherapy Programming in Managed Care Settings

C. Deborah Cross, M.D.

*M*anaged health care has become an increasingly popular concept, particularly with employers concerned about rising health care costs. *Managed health care* is broadly defined as including any form of health care delivery that attempts to control the cost of the service delivered. Initially, this was accomplished through health maintenance organizations (HMOs) in which an organization of physicians and ancillary health care professionals delivered all needed health care for a predetermined, prepaid fee to an identified group of patients. Emphasis was placed on prevention and collaboration. With the apparent initial financial and philosophical success of this new approach, numerous variations began to develop. Terms such as *independent practice association* (IPA) and *preferred provider organization* (PPO) became part of our vocabulary.

A disadvantage of the original HMO concept was patients' lack of choice regarding providers. The newer models sought to overcome this disadvantage by expanding the provider base while initiating cost-control methods such as copayments by patients. Instead of a prepaid fee for overall health care, physicians were recruited to join IPAs and PPOs with the promise of an expanded patient base to offset a negotiated reduction in their standard fee for services. By 1988 there were a total of 734 HMOs and PPOs in the United States, with the majority (456) being IPAs. By 1988, 75% of all California physicians had signed at least one PPO contract and 45% one HMO contract (Herrington 1990).

The development of these and other managed health care models has meant an explosion of growth in patient enrollment. In June of 1992, HMO prepayment plans alone listed an enrollment of 38.8 million people (Hoyt and Austad 1992), and it is estimated that by June 1994, more than 53 million people will be members of managed health care plans (Austad et al. 1992).

The numerous managed health care models share some basic characteristics, including a focus on primary care, control of access to specialists, delivery of cost-effective services with emphasis on office-based practice, use of short-term interventions, and limitation of mental health benefits.

Emphasis in some systems began to be less on prevention and collaboration and more on cost containment. Although mental health care has never achieved reimbursement parity with other areas of health care, the increasing focus on limitation of access to mental health care and curtailment in benefits has been a direct result of increasing concern about costs. The cost of mental health care was easily identifiable and appeared to be increasing at a rate greater than that of the rest of the health care sector (Dickey and Azeni 1992). This situation led to a proliferation of "managed care companies," which marketed their services to insurance companies and employers with a promise to reduce mental health care costs. Insurance companies in turn developed their own managed care subsidiaries and large employers began to use employee assistance programs (EAPs).

Concepts such as precertification of treatment and utilization review have become commonplace. Reimbursement for mental health care treatment can now be denied before being rendered, during the episode of care, or after delivery of the care if the care rendered is deemed to be medically unnecessary or not covered by the patient's insurance by the managed care company. Practitioners are no longer able to assume that they will be reimbursed by insurance for a health care service they perform. As a result, psychiatrists and other mental health care practitioners are increasingly moving away from solo private practice and into group practices (often multidisciplinary) and salary-based positions. In 1980 only 9% of nonfederal psychiatrists were in group practices. In 1988 this number had increased to 15% and it is steadily growing (Council on Long Range Planning and Development 1990).

With psychiatrists and other mental health professionals joining group practices and signing contracts with HMOs and PPOs, the emphasis in treatment has begun to shift away from long-term, individual, insight-oriented psychotherapy. Increasingly, short-term psychotherapies and other nontraditional approaches are being used. Specific schools of short-term psychotherapy have existed since the early 1970s. These approaches have shared an emphasis on brevity, focus, therapist activity, and patient selection (Rutan 1992). However, most mental health practitioners and patients have continued to view short-term psychotherapy as "second best" and philosophically the gold standard of treatment has been non–time-limited psychotherapy.

A review of utilization data suggests that in actual practice "unlimited" psychotherapy is a myth (MacKenzie 1990). The reality is, more often than not, "unplanned" short-term therapy. In most outpatient programs, about two-thirds of the patients are seen for 6 sessions or less, and less than 10% attend for more than 25 sessions (MacKenzie 1990). Another criticism of short-term, time-limited psychotherapy is that patient improvement is jeopardized by such limitation of treatment. Again, objective review of the outcome in outpatient samples appears to prove otherwise. Approximately 50% of patients showed significant improvement by the 8th session and 75% by the 26th session (MacKenzie 1990). Kaiser Permanente in California surveyed 200 patients who were seen for only one visit. Seventy-five percent of the patients reported being "improved" or "much improved" after the one visit and noted their intentions of returning to "their therapist" if the need arose (Schneider-Braus 1992).

Interpretation of such data would seem to indicate that most people who receive mental health treatment do so in a fairly limited number of sessions and that the most improvement in treatment occurs early in the treatment process. Therefore, the long-held assumption by most mental health professionals that unlimited long-term psychotherapy is "better" than and preferable to time-limited psychotherapy does not appear to be warranted.

A similar bias exists toward group psychotherapy, namely that group psychotherapy is second-best, and not as "good" as individual psychotherapy. Again, however, numerous reviews of the data have found that group psychotherapy is as effective as individual treatment and in some specific conditions can have a unique advantage over individual treatment (MacKenzie 1993).

The development of time-limited group psychotherapy is therefore a logical response to the clinical data that show that it is as efficacious as unlimited psychotherapy and as effective as individual psychotherapy. Goals of such time-limited group psychotherapy include symptom reduction, restoration of prior functioning, and effective mobilization of the patient's ego strength. These goals are of course identical in many ways to those stated by the managed mental health care community. In addition, through the group format, these goals can be accomplished in a more cost-effective manner than in individual psychotherapy. Budman (1992) at the Harvard Community Health Plan in Boston has written extensively about brief individual and group psychotherapy models. He has utilized a brief therapy model—"Interpersonal-Developmental-Existential" (IDE)—in which psychotherapy is seen not as a complete "cure," but as an intermittent process throughout the patient's life. Each episode of treatment focuses on why the patient has chosen to seek treatment at that particular time. This approach is also present in Budman's work on time-limited group therapy. In addition, emphasis is placed on establishing a clear and well-defined focus, thoroughly screening and preparing group members, establishing rapid group cohesion, and exploring termination of the specific group relationship.

Although some managed care settings have successfully incorporated group psychotherapy into their programs, many have not. There appears to be a variety of reasons inhibiting the development of successful group psychotherapy programming throughout the managed care field. A fundamental factor is the diversity of practice settings, with the most common remaining the solo practitioner. Training of mental health professionals still focuses predominantly on long-term individual therapeutic models, and the career goal of graduating practitioners continues to be to treat patients in long-term individual psychotherapy in an individual private practice model. Unless practitioners are acquainted and comfortable with short-term and group psychotherapy techniques, they are at a distinct disadvantage in the modern health care field, where the emphasis is increasingly on short-term, cost-effective psychotherapeutic interventions.

Mental health practitioners in group practices often fare little better, because they, too, are at the mercy of their training. Indeed, they often find themselves pushed by administrators to do time-limited therapy, either individual or group, without proper educational preparation or philosophical commitment. Closed-system staff model HMOs appear to have had the most success in incorporating group psychotherapy into their mental health programs. Schneider-Braus (1992) noted that the development of an "underlying shared mission to provide members with quality care in a cost-effective manner" is essential to the effective functioning of such a mental health department in a staff model HMO. Ideally, there should be an "alignment of values" between the insuring organization and the mental health professionals who deliver the services. With this shared basic philosophical mission and commitment, staff members are able to become more flexible and eclectic in their treatment approaches.

Developing a Group Therapy Program

When a mental health organization has a commitment to deliver cost-effective quality mental health care to its patients, the development of a planned and integrated group psychotherapy program should naturally occur. The involvement of administrative personnel throughout the planning process is essential (Folkers and Steefel 1991; MacKenzie 1990) and ensures that appropriate priority is placed on resources, referrals, scheduling, and continuing education. In addition, involvement and commitment of all professional staff is necessary for successful implementation. When the major reason for establishing a group psychotherapy program in an organization is to have clinicians see more patients in less time with little or no concern about staff and patient needs, a recipe for failure exists, with low morale, staff burnout, and patient dissatisfaction.

A carefully thought out, well-researched, and integrated group psychotherapy program is a valuable asset in any mental health care setting. Even a psychiatrist in individual private practice, particularly if he or she is a member of an IPA or a PPO, can develop a well-planned group psychotherapy program that is beneficial and cost-effective to the practitioner, the patient, and the managed health care company. Alternatively, several members of an IPA or a PPO can join together and develop a more elaborate group program structure.

Initial preparation for implementing such a group psychotherapy program within an HMO or other mental health care organization is of critical importance. An organizational retreat where all staff, in an atmosphere of mutual respect, discuss the organization's mission and goals and explore staff roles and attitudes will result in shared owner-ship of and commitment to the task. Most organizations do not have the luxury of recruiting and hiring only those mental health professionals who are well trained in and philosophically committed to brief individ-ual and group psychotherapies. Helping staff make such attitudinal changes is essential. When management simply announces and at-tempts to implement new programs without staff involvement and commitment, failure of the new program usually results.

One of the major benefits that a well-developed group psycho-therapy program offers within a managed care setting is the adaptabil-ity of group psychotherapy to the overall managed care philosophy of intermittent psychotherapy throughout the life cycle (Austad and Hoyt 1992). Because it is expected that the patient will periodically experi-ence crises and disruptions in functioning, utilization of appropriate intermittent group psychotherapy can restore the patient quickly to his or her previous level of functioning with the clear understanding by both patient and therapist that further interventions may be necessary at some future point in the patient's life.

Whether the aim is to establish a comprehensive group psychother-apy program within a clinic or group practice setting or to market a more limited program to managed care companies developed by an individual or small group of practitioners, the primary goal is the same: to deliver clinically needed and relevant group psychotherapy in a cost-effective manner to patients who will most benefit from this therapeutic intervention, either as the only treatment modality or in conjunction with individual treatment.

A survey of the available patient population is a primary requisite, with attention being given to assessment of the varied clinical needs of individual patients. This survey should include basic individual patient data such as diagnostic category, age, sex, marital status, previous treatment (individual and/or group), and current level of functioning for all patients currently in treatment. An overview of the service delivery system is helpful. This should include a review of any new patients awaiting treatment and a compilation of each clinician's caseload with information regarding day and evening schedules, as well as an exam-ination of historical patterns of use by patients of the clinic's services. Decisions regarding whether to treat specific disorders within a group framework can range from very inclusive to more restrictive, reflecting the organizational and staff philosophy.

Once this information has been gathered, the staff can proceed with the development of a group psychotherapy program. At this stage, an understanding of various group psychotherapy models useful in managed care is helpful. Time-limited group psychotherapy models traditionally include a spectrum of groups, ranging from the more supportive to the more psychodynamic; these groups can be categorized as social skills, psychoeducational, interpersonal-restitutive, and interpersonal-explorative (MacKenzie 1993). Social skills groups are helpful for patients who have major difficulties in social functioning. Psychoeducational groups focus on imparting specific information or skills. Interpersonal-restitutive groups help patients cope with specific stressors in their lives. Interpersonal-explorative groups are designed to help patients explore their internal feelings, identify areas of conflict, and use the interpersonal relationships in the group to help them understand the way they relate to people outside the group. Folkers and Steefel (1991) describe a similar series of group models for use in managed care settings. They categorize these models as social skills, psychoeducational, crisis intervention, and developmental stage.

Social Skills Groups

A social skills group is designed to enable people to become more aware of their social behavior and their interactions with others and, by such awareness, to improve their social and work relationships. This model is therefore similar to the traditional social skills model. Providing a safe setting with an imposed social structure and the active support of the group leader allows patients the opportunity to develop new and more appropriate social behaviors, thereby improving their social and work relationships and functioning.

Use of outpatient groups for patients needing this type of intervention can be an alternative to more expensive and disruptive hospitalization. An example of this type of group in an outpatient managed care setting would be a group for patients who have recently been discharged from an inpatient psychiatric unit. In such a group, patients can continue their interpersonal growth, but with a focus on reorientation within the community and adaptation to everyday life.

Psychoeducational Groups

Psychoeducational groups can be effective in imparting skills or information relating to a specific topic. Within managed care settings, particularly HMOs that have as part of their focus a commitment to the prevention of illness, this type of group is readily accepted by both administrators and patients. Examples of this type of group are a parents' group for children with attention-deficit disorder and a group for patients with phobic avoidance disorders who are taught behavioral techniques. Examples of groups that have a purely educational format are a smoking cessation group and a stress management group.

Crisis Intervention Groups

This model is similar to the interpersonal-restitutive model described by MacKenzie (1993), but with a focus on patients in crisis. It is very useful in managed care settings because it allows a clinic or group practice to respond quickly to patients in crisis and thereby prevent clinical deterioration. Often after such therapeutic intervention, further treatment is not clinically indicated or sought by the patient. Because this format is relatively new and offers a way of managing a large volume of patients, it will be described in more detail. Several variations of crisis intervention groups have been described.

New patient referrals. A problem often identified in mental health clinics is the amount of time it takes for a new patient to be seen for an initial appointment. An effective solution is an ongoing brief psychotherapy group for patients new to the clinic. One model for this approach, called "immediate treatment groups," was developed by Lonergan (1985). Patients who request an appointment at the clinic are contacted by one of the group leaders via telephone for initial screening and preparation.

Lonergan (1985) suggested specific screening criteria for entrance into the groups. Patients whose symptoms (e.g., anxiety, depression, somatic complaints) are of acute and recent onset and likely to be resolvable or greatly remediated in a short period of time, as well as patients who present with long-standing masochistic problems even without acute exacerbation, are good candidates for these groups. Patients should not be psychotic or currently suicidal or homicidal. Patients who have histories of previous erratic attendance at the clinic or who have shown little or no change in individual sessions should not be included in these groups.

Specific attention is paid to the patient's resistance to a group format. In Lonergan's model, the group meets weekly, and when a new patient joins the group the expectation is for his or her attendance to be somewhere between 6 and 20 sessions. Lonergan listed five major therapeutic factors in her crisis group model:

1. Emotional catharsis in an accepting and cohesive environment
2. Cognitive understanding of the presenting situation
3. Building self-esteem
4. Optimism about the ability of people to rapidly change
5. Learning to deal with termination

Advantages of such an open group model include having group members at various stages of treatment serve as role models for newer members and the involvement of an active group leader. Modifications of this model include, for example, an initial treatment plan for each new patient with a specified number of group sessions, followed by a review of the patient's progress and recommendations for further treatment if needed. This might involve continuation either within the group or in another treatment setting.

Patients currently being treated in the clinic. Another frequently encountered problem in mental health clinics is that of patients currently in treatment who request emergency appointments. Depending on the extent of the problem and how disruptive such emergency appointments are to the clinic schedule, establishment of crisis or "drop in" groups can be an effective solution. These groups may only be needed weekly (but can be used daily), depending on the clinic's patient population and needs. Patient referral and preparation for the group is accomplished by the patient's clinician and can be done either on the phone or in person. These groups are not appropriate for psychotic or acutely suicidal patients, who should receive other, more appropriate, interventions.

Numerous variations of this model can be developed, depending on the clinic's specific needs. For example, if the clinic treats a large number of patients with borderline personality disorder who experience periodic crises, rather than having each individual therapist schedule emergency appointments as needed with each patient, the clinical option of referral to a crisis group provides a safe and effective treatment plan. Of course, care must be taken to ensure that these referrals are for treatment of crisis situations and do not instead encourage unhealthy dependency by the patient. Other appropriate referrals to this type of a group would include patients who are experiencing an interpersonal crisis (e.g., breakup of a relationship, job termination, death of a relative or friend) that has resulted in a compromised ability to function.

Major catastrophes.   Occasionally, a community experiences a catastrophic event that affects large numbers of its population, including many patients already in treatment at the mental health center. Catastrophic events can range from a devastating fire or other natural disaster to a crime or fatal accident. Survivors and relatives of victims of such a shared traumatic and emotional event often present for mental health treatment. These patients can be very effectively helped by involvement in a group psychotherapy experience. This type of group meets for a specific number of sessions (usually 6–9) with a closed enrollment. An example of this type of group is providing a group psychotherapy experience for teenagers who were present on a school bus when a classmate was accidentally killed.

Developmental Stage Groups

The developmental stage group model allows patients who are similar in age but with heterogeneous initial complaints to be treated in the same group with a focus on shared age-appropriate developmental tasks (Budman et al. 1980). Although this model is similar to the more traditional interpersonal-explorative one, the focus within managed care remains on short-term interventions. Therefore, the developmental stage model focuses on specific age-related themes, stressing normal aspects of development, with the goal of early restoration and improvement of patient functioning. Examples of this type of group include adolescent girls' groups, groups for new parents, and groups for recently retired professionals. All of the group psychotherapy models can be used either as the sole treatment modality for the patient or in conjunction with other psychotherapeutic treatments (e.g., individual psychotherapy or pharmacotherapy). In addition, patients can receive a variety of treatment modalities at various times throughout their lives.

Group Program Management

Once the staff and administration of a mental health organization have decided to implement a group psychotherapy program, have become familiar with the various group models, and have completed a patient-needs survey, the next step is designing an organization-specific program to meet the identified individual patient and overall clinic needs. A sample group psychotherapy program in a medium-sized clinic might include a crisis group set up to triage new patients presenting to the clinic, a women's group focusing on such midlife issues as adult children leaving home, a parents' group for children with attention-deficit disorder, a couples' group for dealing with marital problems, an adolescent girls' group with a focus on interpersonal relations, and an antidepressant medication group for people on maintenance medication. These groups would usually meet for a fixed number of sessions, and new groups would continually be formed as patient needs are identified.

Traditionally, group psychotherapists wait for a specific number of patients with a homogeneous set of needs to begin a new group. This approach to starting a group is counter to that of a managed care setting, where the overall staffing pressures of a clinic require new groups to be started quickly and often with a smaller number of patients. Even a group with four members is more advantageous than treating those four patients individually with consequent loss of staff time. Therefore, conventional conceptions about the size and makeup of groups need to be reexamined in the context of using the group psychotherapy modality in a more varied and utilitarian way.

Staff collaboration, involvement, and commitment are vital ingredients in the development and maintenance of a group psychotherapy program. Although not all of the professional staff can be actively involved in the group psychotherapy program, commitment to the concept of group psychotherapy as a main component of the treatment modalities being offered in the clinic is a necessity for all staff. Therefore, training of all staff in the principles of group psychotherapy is helpful, although comprehensive training of those staff who will be actively involved in the group psychotherapy program is a necessity.

This training is more easily accomplished if the clinic already has one or two well-trained group psychotherapists on staff. If such staff is not available, serious thought should be given to hiring a clinician with appropriate higher-level group and teaching experience. The experienced group psychotherapist can then take a leadership role in developing the overall group program and training new staff. A commitment to training and preparation of staff should eliminate the unfortunate practice of assigning the least well-trained, most junior staff members to lead groups.

Investment by a mental health clinic in adequate training of leaders is cost effective. When a clinic allows untrained or poorly trained clinicians to lead groups, patients do not improve and use more and more costly clinic services. In addition, staff burnout and dissatisfaction occurs as unprepared group leaders struggle to deliver inadequate services. Obviously, the commitment of so much time and energy by staff to establish and maintain a group psychotherapy program must be continually encouraged and supported by the clinic administration. Reference to the shared mission and goals of clinic and staff to provide high-quality, cost-effective treatment is helpful, as well as involvement of the entire professional staff during the development of the program, thereby creating a sense of ownership, support, and acceptance.

Assignment of interested but untrained staff as coleaders of groups can be an effective modality in an overall training process that must also include didactic and other more formal educational methods. As Schneider-Braus (1992) pointed out, setting fair and realistic expectations of the percentage of direct care provided by each clinician is of utmost importance. Allowing clinicians sufficient time for training, continuing education, supervision, and administrative tasks such as record keeping and telephone calls is a priority.

When a group psychotherapy program is implemented, attention must also be paid to record keeping and communication. Any time a patient receives treatment from more than one provider, communication between clinicians is vital. This is particularly true in a clinic setting, where patients routinely are seen by many different providers (e.g., by on-call clinicians). This type of communication can be verbal; however, record keeping is still a necessity, for both ethical and legal reasons. In addition, utilization review standards usually require a note in each patient's chart for each service provided. Ideally, each patient should have an individualized note for each group session he or she attended. However, this is often quite impractical. A form for a group progress note can be developed in which general group information such as date, number of attendees, central issue(s) of the session, and plans for future session are recorded. On individual copies of this form, personalized information such as the patient's name, medications (if any), and current mental status can be recorded.

A clinic may decide that it is acceptable for a group clinician to write a general group therapy note for each session and then have this note put in each attending patient's chart. Alternatively, if the group has a specified number of sessions, the expectation can be to have only a termination note in each group member's chart. The balance between charting requirements, communication between providers, and patient confidentiality is unique to each mental health clinic setting but must be established when the group program is designed and then adhered to by all clinicians.

Just as clinic staff need preparation for a group psychotherapy program, so too do patients. Many patients need education regarding basic techniques of psychotherapy such as introspection, self-disclosure, and focus on feelings. Also, patients need to be introduced to the concept of group psychotherapy and the benefits such treatment can afford them. A formal brief pregroup preparation period is necessary for patients who have not been involved in group psychotherapy. This can be useful, as well, for patients who have participated in group therapy but who may need some refocusing and retraining in group process. Such preparation can be done in either individual or group sessions; studies indicate that preparation results in fewer early dropouts (MacKenzie 1993). Pregroup preparation allows the clinician to screen out the patients who are inappropriate for the group or who need another type of treatment. It also enables the clinician to make sure that all patients are aware of the "rules" of group participation, such as regular attendance, notification in advance of absences and termination, confidentiality, focus on feelings, and verbal participation.

Patient resistance to group psychotherapy is a major focus of pregroup preparation. The clinician should expect the patient to be anxious about entering a group experience and to insist instead on individual psychotherapy. A matter-of-fact and informative approach in which the clinician says, "The best treatment for your problem is group therapy," and then tells the patient when the specific group meets often helps a great deal in defusing such resistance. In addition, the clinician should reassure the patients that their anxiety about being in a group is a very normal reaction and that, in fact, group therapy is especially helpful for people who have trouble speaking up in front of others. The clinician should explain that group therapy offers the opportunity to get feedback from other people who are struggling with the same types of problems.

It is helpful to provide the patient with some specific suggestions during the pregroup preparation about how to deal with anxiety during the first session. This might include encouraging the patient to verbalize feelings (e.g., "I'm feeling anxious about being here") or to comment on what other group members talk about (Lonergan 1985). When pregroup preparation is done in a group setting, MacKenzie (1990) has suggested using structured group exercises as an educational tool. An example is to have members identify something they would like to change or better understand in a personal relationship. Good pregroup preparation promotes rapid group cohesion, which is a necessity in time-limited group psychotherapy. With staff and patients knowledgeable of and committed to an ongoing group psychotherapy program, referrals of patients and establishment of new groups will become an accepted part of the overall treatment planning within the clinic.

With a clear commitment by the clinic or group practice to group psychotherapy as a major treatment modality, the clinic is able to present its comprehensive group psychotherapy program to managed care companies as a favorable option for patient referrals. Managed care companies are interested in cost-effective and easily implemented treatment plans. By providing access to a diverse cross-section of time-limited and focused groups to which managed care companies can easily refer patients for treatment, a clinic or group practice is well placed for participation in the evolving mental health care arena. A smaller clinic or group practice can decide to specialize in only some of the groups outlined above (e.g., medication groups, parent groups, or women's groups) and offer their expertise to managed care companies for specialized patient referrals.

The challenge that faces all mental health care providers today is to provide treatment that is both beneficial and cost effective. A well-planned group psychotherapy program gives practitioners many options to meet both goals. It should therefore be a part of any practitioner's or clinic's array of psychotherapeutic interventions.

References

Austad CS, Hoyt MF: The managed care movement and the future of psychotherapy. Psychotherapy 29:109–118, 1992

Austad CS, Sherman WO, Morgan T, et al: The psychotherapist and the managed care setting. Professional Psychology: Research and Practice 23:329–332, 1992

Budman SH: Models of brief individual and group psychotherapy, in Managed Mental Health Care. Edited by Feldman J, Fitzpatrick R. Washington, DC, American Psychiatric Press, 1992, pp 231–248

Budman SH, Bennett MJ, Wisnecki MJ: Short-term group psychotherapy: an adult developmental model. Int J Group Psychother 30:63–76, 1980

Council on Long Range Planning and Development: Council report: the future of psychiatry. JAMA 264:2542–2548, 1990

Dickey B, Azeni H: Impact of managed care on mental health services. Health Affairs 11:197–204, 1992

Folkers CE, Steefel NM: Group psychotherapy, in Psychotherapy in Managed Health Care. Edited by Austad CS, Berman WH. Washington, DC, American Psychological Association, 1991, pp 46–64

Herrington BS: Independent practice associations mushroom as physicians scramble to join. Psychiatric News 25(5):14, March 2, 1990

Hoyt MF, Austad CS: Psychotherapy in a staff model health maintenance organization: Providing and assuring quality care in the future. Psychotherapy 29:119–128, 1992

Lonergan E: Utilizing group process in crisis-waiting-list groups. Int J Group Psychother 35:355–372, 1985

MacKenzie KR: Introduction to Time-Limited Group Psychotherapy. Washington, DC, American Psychiatric Press, 1990

MacKenzie KR: Time-limited group therapy and technique, in Group Therapy in Clinical Practice. Edited by Alonso A, Swiller H. Washington, DC, American Psychiatric Press, 1993, pp 423–447

Rutan JS: Psychotherapy for the 1990s. New York, Guilford, 1992

Schneider-Braus K: Managing a mental health department in a staff model HMO, in Managed Mental Health Care. Edited by Feldman J, Fitzpatrick R. Washington, DC, American Psychiatric Press, 1992, pp 125–142

Chapter 3

Brief Intensive Group Psychotherapy for Loss

William E. Piper, Ph.D.

*E*scalating costs for health care suggest that the adoption of some form of managed care is necessary. This is probably the case whether the administrative structures are part of governments, health care organizations, insurance companies, or other types of third-party payment sources. However, regardless of the apparent appropriateness of managed care, a number of serious concerns have arisen. Consumers fear that the quality of health care will be sacrificed as the result of single-minded efforts to contain costs. Practitioners fear that their professional autonomy and judgment will be usurped by rigid administrative policies. Private third-party sources fear that their efforts to implement managed care may generate so much criticism that governments will be forced to create parallel structures that eventually will put them out of business. Thus, managed care is viewed by all of the major parties involved as having the potential for substantial negative, as well as positive, consequences. Evidence of successful clinical programs that are compatible with managed care may serve to lessen some of the concerns. In this chapter, I present evidence of such a program.

In the mental health field, high costs are associated with the entire range of treatment services. These include full-time hospitalization, partial hospitalization, and outpatient treatment. Some administrators have identified the treatment of certain patient groups (e.g., substance abuse patients and disturbed adolescents) as being a particularly heavy drain on health care budgets (Welch 1992). Questions have been raised about the necessity of full-time hospitalization for these patients. Similarly, questions have been raised about the necessity of providing continual day-care services for chronic, low-functioning psychiatric patients (Hoge et al. 1992). In the area of outpatient treatment, the need to provide multiple sessions per week or long-term therapy (or both) for moderately disturbed patients has been debated for many years. For psychosocial interventions such as outpatient psychotherapy, a logical solution would seem to be a greater use of time-limited therapies of short-term duration—in particular, group therapies.

However, just as the idea of managed care has generated serious concern among many practitioners, so too has the idea of providing time-limited, short-term group therapies. Part of the concern is based on legitimate doubts about the effectiveness of time-limited group therapies because of their salient structural differences compared with open-ended individual therapies. Practitioners raise the obvious question, "What can be accomplished for my patient in a group that lasts only a short time?" Another source of concern stems from the fact that many practitioners are less comfortable in the role of group therapist than in the role of individual therapist. Facing a group of patients is generally more anxiety arousing than facing a single patient in treatment.

Unfortunately, the training and experience of many therapists have not prepared them for providing group therapy, let alone time-limited, short-term group therapy. If therapists do not feel at ease in conducting group therapy, it is not surprising that they do not readily embrace it. In addition, groups are more complicated to organize. An entire set of patients must be assembled to begin at the same time. If one or more patients falter, the onset of the entire group can be affected, as well as its viability. Another factor that should not be overlooked is that, when asked, most patients indicate a preference for individual treatment. Thus, reluctance on the therapist's part is frequently reinforced by reluctance on the patients' part. For all of these reasons, the notion of time-limited, short-term group therapy as a solution to problems related to managed care is questionable to many practitioners.

To address the reservations of practitioners, two types of information are particularly relevant. The first is evidence that time-limited, short-term group therapy works; this concerns benefit to patients. The second is evidence that programs that offer this type of therapy work; this concerns benefit to practitioners. There is a growing body of scientific evidence that attests to the comparable efficacy of group and individual therapies. Much of the evidence is summarized in literature reviews of controlled and comparative studies of group and individual therapies (Robinson et al. 1990; Smith et al. 1980; Tillitski 1990; Toseland and Siporin 1986). In addition, reports of new studies appear regularly in the literature. Many of the group therapies studied have homogeneous patient compositions and are of short-term duration. Patients with a variety of disorders are treated, including patients with eating disorders (Wilfley et al. 1993), parasuicidal patients with border-line personality disorder (Linehan et al. 1991), patients with chronic back pain (Turner et al. 1990), patients with avoidant personality disorders (Alden 1989), female incest survivors (Alexander et al. 1989), patients with major depression (Rehm et al. 1987), cancer patients (Telch and Telch 1986), and depressed adolescents (Reynolds and Coats 1986).

Reports of success with time-limited, short-term group therapies can be persuasive, especially if practitioners are involved in the treatment of the patient populations that are described in published studies. However, reports of patient benefits usually do not address the second type of information—practitioner benefits. Practitioners may wonder whether the therapists who provided the treatment found the experience stimulating and gratifying. Was there much enthusiasm among staff? Was there staff attrition? Did the program that sponsored the groups continue after the study was completed? Or did the program atrophy and cease after the study? Would something similar occur as a result of a managed care initiative? Evidence of benefit to practitioners may be just as important as evidence of benefit to patients in diminishing resistance and promoting interest in group-oriented managed care.

Loss Group Program

Since 1986 we have conducted a program for treating psychiatric outpatients who have experienced difficulty adapting to the loss of one or more persons (Piper et al. 1992). The treatment modality was time-limited, short-term group psychotherapy. Since the onset of the program, more than 30 groups have been completed. The first 16 groups were studied as part of a controlled clinical trial to evaluate the effectiveness of the treatment approach. The subsequent 14 groups were conducted as part of the ongoing treatment program. Our experience provided evidence of both treatment efficacy (patient benefit) and program efficacy (practitioner benefit). We believe that the program is representative of the type that can be successfully implemented as part of a managed care approach to mental health service delivery.

Setting and Motivating Factors

The Loss Group Program is situated within the Walk-In Clinic at the Division of External Psychiatric Services of the University of Alberta Hospitals. The division is a large, multifaceted outpatient service for psychiatric patients that is located within an 800-bed university hospital. The catchment area includes Edmonton, a city of approximately 700,000, and the surrounding region, which includes an additional 500,000 people. The walk-in clinic is a high-volume service that handles approximately 2,400 initial assessments each year. A variety of treatment alternatives, including individual, couple, family, and group therapy; psychopharmacology; and partial hospitalization, are regularly provided.

A survey conducted in 1986 as part of a routine service evaluation revealed that many of the patients in the clinic suffered from unresolved reactions to loss of a loved one or friend. The findings of the survey led to the idea of creating a special program to serve these patients' needs. A review of the literature concerning short-term individual therapies and group therapies suggested that a focused approach with a time limit and a homogeneous patient composition would be useful. What emerged was a model for conducting time-limited, short-term therapy groups for these patients. A pilot program involving a small number of staff was started. Its success led to a proposal for a more formalized program that was accepted by the clinic staff. Although the program did not result from a centralized managed care initiative, the motivating factors were similar. These included a large demand for services, limited resources, and the prospect of a cost-effective method of treatment.

Procedures and Staff

The Loss Group Program was designed to provide patients with a short-term group form of treatment, and therapists with an opportunity to learn about the topic of loss and how to treat patients with problems related to loss. The loss groups represented a treatment alternative for the 15 walk-in clinic therapists and 6 supervisory psychiatrists who routinely conduct initial assessments. Because patients coming to the clinic rarely present with a self-diagnosis of pathological grief, the assessors must be familiar with indications and risk factors associated with pathological grief. When a patient is judged to be suitable, he or she is referred to a program coordinator who serves as a liaison between patients waiting for a group and therapists waiting to conduct a group. Once presented with a set of patients, the therapist informs them about the starting date of the group and makes arrangements for its onset. New patients are sometimes added through the second session. In the case of the groups in the research project, the assessment and preparation activities were somewhat more complicated; they are described below.

The therapists of the groups are a multidisciplinary team of nonmedical professionals from the disciplines of psychology, social work, nursing, and occupational therapy. All participate in a weekly, 1-hour seminar led by the clinical psychologist who is director of the program. The seminar serves a number of clinical, academic, and administrative purposes. However, the mainstay activity of the seminar is listening to recordings of loss group sessions and discussing issues related to the selection, preparation, and treatment of patients. Thus, the focus of the seminar remains close to the clinical material. Discussion of articles from the literature and construction of a demonstration videotape are additional activities that take place during the seminar. Supervision for specific groups is conducted outside the seminar. In general, the seminar serves as a vehicle for strengthening the cohesion and morale of the treatment team. This function is viewed as essential because of the demanding task of conducting short-term loss groups.

Therapy

The conceptual and technical orientation of therapy is psychodynamic—that is, based on the idea that recurrent internal conflicts whose components are largely unconscious serve to perpetuate maladaptation. Conflicts concerning the issues of intimacy versus isolation and independence versus dependence in the context of loss are common in this patient population. The general objective of therapy is to help patients solve their presenting problems by achieving insight into how their difficulties are related to unresolved intrapsychic conflicts and by initiating a process of working through that continues beyond the treatment sessions. More specific objectives include the following:

1. Diminished intensity of symptoms associated with loss
2. Greater tolerance of ambivalent feelings toward lost persons
3. Insight into long-standing conflicts that have contributed to unsatisfactory relationships
4. Adaptive steps toward achieving gratifying relationships and productive performance in other areas

The groups meet once a week for 90 minutes for 12 weeks. Their technical orientation includes an active therapist whose role it is to emphasize interpretation and clarification in relationship to support and direction. Relevant here-and-now events in the group, including transference, are highlighted and examined. As a composite illustration, consider the following interchange. The therapist had just drawn the absence of one of the patients (Ellen) to the group's attention and suggested that they might be feeling responsible or guilty.

Sarah: [interrupting] I think it was just too much for Ellen, hearing everything, like when I was talking about my mother. She was really upset, you could just tell, you know. But she couldn't say anything. Then when she started crying, I thought, well, I guess, yeah, I thought you [the therapist] maybe should do something, like to calm her down, so she wouldn't feel so bad.

Kyle: Or maybe you [the therapist] should have stayed with her after group and not just stopped it right at 11:30.

Sarah: Yeah, I kinda wondered about that too, you know.

Alice: [interrupting] Well, I think she [the therapist] wouldn't be running the group if she, you know, she must know how you're supposed to do it, you know, get on with your life.

Margaret: Well, I think Ellen was overwhelmed by what I said. You know, I was kind of upset and maybe said too much.

Michel: I don't think it makes a difference how we feel about Helen [sic]. I'm upset about my wife, not some stranger.

Margaret: Yeah, I feel sort of annoyed, or frustrated with you [the therapist] 'cause how can you feel bad about losing someone you never even got to know?

Lois: I think we need to get to know how to stop dwelling on the past, like how do we stop feeling like this.

Therapist: So there are some mixed feelings about me. There is some disappointment that I didn't take care of Ellen better, calm her down; that I point out that you may have some feelings about her not being here today. And there's the hope that I really do know what I'm doing, that I am going to help you.

Thus, after listening to how the group responded to her comment about the missing member, the therapist chose to address their conflictual feelings (disappointment, hope) about her (the therapist). This was consistent with the approach of exploring conflictual feelings (guilt, anger) about one another (e.g., Ellen, people in their lives whom they had lost). In a more supportive form of group therapy, the therapist might have reassured the members about their guilt concerning Ellen and accentuated the positive feelings they had about her (the therapist).

Two additional technical features guide the therapist: consistent focus on commonalities and use of structural limitations. *Commonalities* are the characteristics that patients share. These include the historical events of loss, symptomatology/dysfunction, long-standing conflicts, and experiences in the group. The commonalities allow the therapist to effectively involve most if not all of the patients through group interpretations. *Structural limitations* refer to the group format and limited time.

The challenge is to transform these potential liabilities into assets. Limited possibilities for individual attention in the group create opportunities to examine dependency needs. Absenteeism and dropping out, as illustrated above, create opportunities to reexamine reactions to lost persons in the present situation. The limited time associated with the group creates opportunities to examine existential concerns regarding limitations in life and the inevitability of loss. The following example demonstrates how even in the very first session the therapist may want to remind the group about the time limit of the group and its implications. This intervention followed a period when efforts at making initial introductions appeared to be slowing down.

Therapist: There seems to be some reluctance to get beyond the brief introductions that have been made. I wonder if that is related to the difficult challenge you face—of opening up and sharing your experiences with loss when you all know that in only 12 weeks you will lose each other.

This interpretation has multiple implications. It is one way that the therapist can use the structural limitations of the group to further the patients' understanding of their experiences with loss and how those experiences continue to affect them.

Evaluation of Treatment Effectiveness

The first 16 groups of the program were studied in a controlled clinical trial (Piper et al. 1992). After providing informed consent, patients participated in a 3-hour assessment that included interview and questionnaire measures. The assessment provided initial scores for the personality variable, psychological mindedness, and a number of outcome variables. Psychological mindedness was viewed as potentially important to treatment outcome. Patients were matched in pairs on psychological mindedness, gender, and age, and randomly assigned to an immediate treatment or a control (delayed treatment) group. Therapists were assigned a matched pair of groups (one immediate, one delayed); there were eight matched pairs in the trial. Each group contained patients who were high and who were low on psychological mindedness. Outcome variables were reassessed after treatment and the control period, and at follow-up 6 months after completion of treatment.

Patients

A total of 154 patients completed their initial assessments and were assigned to either an immediate treatment or a control group. A number of patients dropped out at various times during the study. Some patients (decliners) changed their minds before starting therapy; others (therapy dropouts) began therapy but left prematurely, i.e., before their group ended (30%). Ambivalence about beginning and continuing is common in therapy groups, and short-term loss groups are no exception.

For the outcome analyses that compared patients in the immediate treatment groups with patients in the control groups, 94 patients (42 immediate patients, 52 delay patients) provided pre- and postoutcome data. The sample of 94 consisted of 68 women and 26 men. Their average age was 36.0 years. Over two-thirds (68%) of the patients did not live with a partner, being widowed (14%), separated (13%), divorced (21%), or single (20%). Most (85%) had a least a high school education, whereas over a quarter (29%) had attended or were attending a technical college and almost one-third (32%) had attended or were attending a university. Most (80%) of the patients were employed, responsible for a household, or involved in studies.

All patients were assessed as experiencing a pathological grief reaction following the loss of a person through death (29%), separation/divorce (12%), or both types of losses (59%). Their most recent loss had occurred a minimum of 3 months before referral to the program.

In terms of DSM-III (American Psychiatric Association 1980), the most common diagnoses were major depression (45%), adjustment disorder (16%), dysthymia (10%), and anxiety disorder (9%). Fourteen percent also received an Axis II diagnosis, usually dependent disorder (11%). Patients manifesting problems of suicidal intent, psychosis, addiction, sexual deviation, sociopathic behavior, or who were currently involved in another form of psychotherapy were excluded from the study. Sixty-nine percent of the patients had previous contact with a mental health professional, but only 11% had previously received psychotherapy. Interviews with patients after the immediate treatment or delay period revealed that 46% had taken psychotropic medication during the initial 3-month period of the study. In almost all cases (95%), it involved antidepressant medication.

Balance Between Conditions

Before making outcome comparisons between immediate treatment and control patients, and between patients high and low on psychological mindedness, the patients in the two treatment conditions were examined to see if they were balanced on six types of potentially confounding variables. These included demographic characteristics, diagnoses, loss characteristics, initial levels of disturbance, medications, and other psychotherapies. There were no significant differences between patients in the immediate treatment and control conditions, nor between patients high and low on psychological mindedness on any of the variables, thus indicating a high degree of balance.

Outcome Variables

The areas represented in the battery of outcome variables (Table 3–1) included interpersonal functioning, psychiatric symptomatology, self-

Table 3–1.   Outcome measures and variables

Measure	Variables
Social Adjustment Scale interview (Weissman et al. 1971)	Work area; social area; family-of-origin area; sexual area
Interpersonal Dependency Inventory (Hirshfield et al. 1977)	Emotional reliance; autonomy
Interpersonal Behavior Scale (Piper et al. 1977)	Present functioning; present–ideal discrepancy
Symptom Checklist–90 (Derogatis 1977)	Global severity index
Beck Depression Inventory (Beck and Steer 1987)	Depression
Impact of Events Scale (Horowitz et al. 1979)	Intrusion; avoidance
Rosenberg Self-Esteem Scale (Rosenberg 1979)	Self-esteem
Life-Satisfaction Scale (Piper et al. 1992)	Life satisfaction
Target objectives	Severity rated by patient; severity rated by independent assessor

esteem, life satisfaction, and personalized target objectives. The sources of evaluation included the patient and an independent assessor.

Outcome Findings

Given the large number of outcome variables assessed, a multivariate analysis was conducted initially. The two-by-two multivariate analysis of variance (MANOVA), which was used with residual gain scores, examined the main effect of treatment, the main effect of psychological mindedness, and the interaction effect. Only the main effect for treatment was significant (Pillais F [16,48] = 2.09, $P < .03$); therefore, only univariate effects for treatment were explored (Table 3–2). For each of the 10 significant variables, treated patients improved more than control patients.

In contrast to statistical significance, the criterion known as *magnitude of effect* directly expresses the size of impact that one variable has on another—in our case, treatment on outcome. We calculated

Table 3–2. Treatment main effects for 16 outcome variables

Outcome variable	n	F
Work area (SAS)	79	2.22
Social area (SAS)	89	0.02
Family area (SAS)	88	3.40
Sexual area (SAS)	88	4.61[*]
Emotional reliance	87	0.02
Autonomy	87	1.47
Present interpersonal	88	4.84[*]
Present–ideal discrepancy	87	2.76
Global severity index	82	13.07[***]
Depression	88	12.92[***]
Intrusion	87	4.16[*]
Avoidance	87	9.69[**]
Self-esteem	85	12.07[***]
Life satisfaction	73	9.43[**]
Target severity (patient)	82	7.28[**]
Target severity (independent assessor)	87	9.43[**]

Note. SAS = Social Adjustment Scale (Weissman et al. 1971).
[*]$P < .05$.
[**]$P < .01$.
[***]$P < .001$.

magnitude of effect according to the formula provided by Smith et al. (1980): magnitude of effect is the difference in average outcome between treated patients and control patients divided by the standard deviation of the control patients. All the effect sizes were positive in sign, indicating greater benefit for treated patients. The average effect size for all 16 variables was 0.51. The average effect size for the 10 variables that had significant treatment effects was 0.67. Such effect sizes are usually regarded as moderate to large in the psychotherapy literature. Using the language of Smith and co-workers, an effect size of 0.67 indicates that the benefits of the average treated patient exceeded those of 75% of the control patients.

Clinical significance refers to the clinical importance of an effect. Central to its meaning is the consideration of norms. If a patient moves from a pathological level to a normal level on a particular variable, a clinically significant change has occurred. Norms were available for two of the outcome variables in the study. For the Symptom Checklist–90 (SCL-90), Derogatis (1977) reported a global severity index mean of 1.26 for 1,002 psychiatric outpatients and a mean of 0.31 for 974 nonpatients. Patients in the immediate condition moved from a mean initial level of 1.28 to a posttherapy level of 0.66. Thus, they moved about two-thirds of the way from the psychiatric outpatient level to the nonpatient level. In contrast, control patients moved from a similar mean initial level of 1.36 to a postdelay level of only 1.01, or about one-third of the way toward the nonpatient norm.

For the Beck Depression Inventory, Beck and Steer (1987) reported a mean of 17.5 for 99 dysthymic patients and a mean of 4.7 for 143 female college students. Patients in the immediate condition moved from a mean initial level of 17.6 to a posttherapy level of 8.0, whereas patients in the control condition moved from a mean initial level of 20.1 to a mean postdelay level of 14.4. For both of the variables, it was evident that treated patients did not completely reach the mean levels of untreated patients by the end of their 3-month loss groups. Nevertheless, they came considerably closer than patients in the control condition.

Patient cooperation in providing 6-month follow-up data was excellent. Assessments were available for 90% (68 out of 76) of the patients who had completed either immediate or delayed therapy. Four of the variables (work and social functioning according to the Social Adjustment Scale [Weissman et al. 1971], and emotional reliance and intrusion) showed significant additional improvement over the follow-up period and two of the variables (avoidance and target objective severity rated by the patient) showed nearly significant additional improvement (Table 3–3). The overall pattern of the 16 outcome variables indicated additional improvement or maintenance of benefits 6 months after therapy had ended.

The results of the clinical trial were clearly supportive of the effectiveness of the groups. Treated patients improved significantly more on a number of outcome variables than their matched control counterparts. Some variables were particularly relevant to the problems of loss patients; these included depression, low self-esteem, and the intrusion and avoidance of thoughts about the lost person(s), as well as specific target objectives of the patients. Although most of the outcome

Table 3–3.   Posttherapy to follow-up effects for 16 outcome variables

Outcome variable	n	t
Work area (SAS)	58	2.47[**]
Social area (SAS)	63	2.08[**]
Family area (SAS)	62	1.35
Sexual area (SAS)	63	−0.27
Emotional reliance	66	3.51[***]
Autonomy	66	−0.13
Present interpersonal	66	−0.43
Present–ideal discrepancy	66	0.78
Global severity index	65	0.26
Depression	64	−0.03
Intrusion	61	3.67[***]
Avoidance	61	1.95[*]
Self-esteem	65	1.61
Life satisfaction	57	0.61
Target severity (patient)	82	1.88[*]
Target severity (independent assessor)	87	0.73

Note.   SAS = Social Adjustment Scale (Weissmann et al. 1971).
[*]$P < .10$.
[**]$P < .05$.
[***]$P < .001$.

variables changed more significantly as a result of treatment, not all did. Interpersonal functioning with work associates, friends, and close associates, as well as general interpersonal dependency, did not. It is possible that these variables require a longer course of treatment than 3 months or a different type of therapy. Follow-up assessments suggested that therapeutic processes continued beyond the termination of the therapy groups.

Outcome was also measured in terms of magnitude of effect. The effect sizes ranged from moderate to large and were comparable in size to those reported in meta-analytic reviews of psychotherapy outcome. Examination of the clinical significance of the results for two outcome variables that had normative data indicated important changes for the treated patients. Considering the strengths of the methodology for the clinical trial, we believe that the results provided a strong endorsement for the treatment.

Continuation of the Therapy Groups and Seminar

Since completion of the last (16th) group in the research project (September 1989), 14 additional groups have been conducted for a total of 30 groups in just over 6 years. The total number of patients starting in the groups was 224, which represents an average of 7.5 patients per group. The dropout rate for starters was 26%, or about two patients per group. Thus, approximately three-quarters of the patients starting completed their groups. The conducting of nearly five groups per year represents a significant service component for the clinic.

The loss group seminar has continued on a weekly basis during the 9 academic months (September–May) of each year. The current year's membership is representative. It includes nine psychologists, a social worker, a nurse, an occupational therapist, and a research assistant. The seminar has been well attended and has served as a central communication medium for those involved in the loss group program. The role required of the therapist in a loss group is a demanding one. The therapist must maintain an active presence largely through interpretive rather than supportive techniques. Repeatedly confronting patients with conflictual material often engenders resistance. The material that is discussed is usually associated with negative affects. Direct expressions of appreciation from patients for one's role are infrequent. Thus, the role of the loss group therapist is an energy-consuming one that at times can be stressful. The seminar has provided a useful outlet for discussing the pressures associated with being a therapist in a loss group. In addition to support, the seminar has provided an opportunity for learning as well as a representation of membership in a valued clinical program in our setting.

Consideration of Cost in Terms of Therapist Time

It is possible to compare the average amount of therapist time allocated to each patient in a loss group with the average amount of therapist time allocated to a patient in individual therapy. Based on an average of

7.5 patients in a group for twelve 90-minute sessions, the average time per patient is 2.4 hours. Based on one patient in individual therapy for twelve 45-minute sessions, the average time per patient is 9.0 hours. The ratio is approximately one to four. This means that about four times as many patients can be treated in a group therapy program. If the seminar time of 1 hour per week is also included in the calculations, about twice as many patients can still be treated in a group therapy program. On this basis, loss groups appear to be efficient as well as effective.

Conclusions

If one were asked to select a form of psychotherapy that is maximally economical in terms of therapist time, time-limited, short-term group therapy would be the obvious choice. The prospect of simultaneously treating an entire group of patients in a brief period of time is clearly appealing on economic grounds. Given the recent recessionary economic climate and pressure to adopt some form of managed care, time-limited, short-term group therapy is a logical solution. However, on emotional grounds it often is not. On the one hand, budgetary pressures and administrative directives carry a great deal of weight in clinics and institutions. On the other hand, factors in addition to economic benefit are also very influential.

One factor is the clinical usefulness of the technique. If practitioners are convinced that certain problems are ideally suited to time-limited, short-term therapy, the chances that they will use it are greatly enhanced. Other factors include the degree to which therapists feel comfortable in providing group therapy and the degree to which patients feel satisfied in receiving it. Although research demonstrations of cost-effectiveness are needed, evidence of satisfying clinical experiences with the technique is also needed. Otherwise, time-limited, short-term group therapy runs the risk of being regarded as a second- or third-rate form of treatment that must be endured until the economic climate changes.

The evidence provided in this chapter suggests that time-limited, short-term group therapy may be a treatment of choice for psychiatric patients with pathological grief reactions. The evidence also suggests that it can be a stimulating and gratifying form of treatment for practitioners. Participation in an ongoing seminar appears to be an important contributor to such a benefit. There are a variety of patient problems that can be addressed with time-limited, short-term group therapy. New programs can be started and studied. It is hoped that clinicians and researchers will continue to explore the possibilities of time-limited, short-term group therapy as a treatment of choice and as a response to managed care.

References

Alden L: Short-term structured treatment for avoidant personality disorder. J Consul Clin Psychol 57:756–764, 1989

Alexander PC, Neimeyer RA, Follette VM, et al: A comparison of group treatment of women sexually abused as children. J Consul Clin Psychol 57:479–483, 1989

American Psychiatric Association: Diagnostic and Statistical Manual of Mental Disorders, 3rd Edition. Washington, DC, American Psychiatric Association, 1980

Beck AT, Steer RA: Beck Depression Inventory Manual. New York, Harcourt Brace Jovanovich, 1987

Derogatis LR: SCL–90 Administration, Scoring and Procedures Manual: I. Baltimore, MD, Johns Hopkins University Press, 1977

Hirshfield RMA, Klerman G, Gough H, et al: A measure of interpersonal dependency. J Pers Assess 41:610–618, 1977

Hoge MA, Davidson L, Hill WL, et al: The promise of partial hospitalization: a reassessment. Hosp Community Psychiatry 43:345–354, 1992

Horowitz MJ, Wilner N, Alvarez W: Impact of event scale: a measure of subjective stress. Psychosom Med 41: 209–218, 1979

Linehan MM, Armstrong HE, Suarez A, et al: Cognitive-behavioral treatment of chronically parasuicidal borderline patients. Arch Gen Psychiatry 48:1060–1064, 1991

Piper WE, Debbane EG, Garant J: An outcome study of group therapy. Arch Gen Psychiatry 34:1027–1032, 1977

Piper WE, McCallum M, Azim HFA: Adaptation to Loss Through Short-term Group Psychotherapy. New York, Guilford, 1992

Rehm LP, Kaslow NJ, Rabin AS: Cognitive and behavioral targets in a self-control therapy program for depression. J Consul Clin Psychol 55:60–67, 1987

Reynolds WM, Coats KI: A comparison of cognitive-behavioral therapy and relaxation training for the treatment of depression in adolescents. J Consult Clin Psychol 54:653–660, 1986

Robinson LA, Berman JS, Neimeyer RA: Psychotherapy for the treatment of depression: a comprehensive review of controlled outcome research. Psychol Bull 108:30–49, 1990

Rosenberg M: Conceiving the Self. New York, Basic Books, 1979

Smith MH, Glass GV, Miller TI: The Benefits of Psychotherapy. Baltimore, MD, Johns Hopkins University Press, 1980

Telch CF, Telch MJ: Group coping skills instruction and supportive group therapy for cancer patients: a comparison of strategies. J Consult Clin Psychol 54:802–808, 1986

Tillitski CJ: A meta-analysis of estimated effect size for group vs. individual vs. control treatments. Int J Group Psychother 40:215–224, 1990

Toseland RW, Siporin M: When to recommend group treatment: a review of the clinical and the research literature. Int J Group Psychother 36:171–201, 1986

Turner JA, Clancy S, McQuade KJ, et al: Effectiveness of behavioral therapy for chronic low back pain: a component analysis. J Consult Clin Psychol 58:573–579, 1990

Weissman MM, Paykel ES, Siegal R, et al: The social role performance of depressed women: a comparison with a normal sample. Am J Orthopsychiatry 41:390–405, 1971

Welch BL: Managing managed care: Paradigm I, II and beyond: can psychology survive another 100 years? Practitioner 5:1–11, 1992

Wilfley DE, Agras WS, Telch CF: Group cognitive-behavioral therapy and group interpersonal psychotherapy for the nonpurging bulimic individual: a controlled comparison. J Consult Clin Psychol 61:296–305, 1993

Chapter 4

Structured Groups for the Treatment of Depression

Angie H. Rice, M.S.W., M.Ed.

*I*n an age of increasing economic constriction, managed care, and heightened demands for effectiveness and efficiency by patients and third-party payers, clinicians are challenged to develop creative models for ameliorating the myriad of problems for which people seek help. In this chapter I address one model that integrates a number of theoretical and practice orientations into a unified approach using the interactional framework of the small psychotherapy group to help members achieve their goals in dealing with depression. This program was first developed as an 8-week group for the treatment of depression with patients of a private, nonprofit psychotherapy center. It was modified into a 12-week program for use with patients in a community mental health center. These patients can be identified as constituting a more dysfunctional population, or at least one with a broader range of functionality and with varying degrees and chronicity of depression.

The program strives to efficiently address the treatment needs of a rapidly expanding population of individuals, many with limited financial and personal resources, who exhibit depressive symptoms and illness. It applies a growing body of literature on the successful treatment of depression and incorporates material that has empirical validation. This model can be termed a "multimethod group therapy" approach (Rose 1989).

Extensive personality change or reconstruction is not a realistic goal for any short-term therapy, nor is complete symptom remission.

I wish to acknowledge the assistance of Beverly Woodbury, Tulane M.S.W. student, in the research and design of this model.

Most people come to therapy to deal with a current life problem, precipitated either by a crisis or by an exacerbation of an existing problem by environmental factors. Klein (1985) described therapeutic goals as typically including 1) reducing symptomatic discomfort; 2) fostering a return to the patient's previous emotional equilibrium; 3) promoting efficient use of the patient's resources (e.g., increasing the patient's sense of control or mastery, encouraging adaptation and behavioral change, aiding cognitive restructuring, self-help, and social effectiveness); and 4) developing the patient's understanding of the current disturbance and increasing his or her coping skills.

Selection

Rapid early assessment of the patient's difficulties, capacities, and motivation to engage in therapy is important in order to determine suitability for treatment and facilitate the adoption of appropriate treatment goals (Garvin 1990). The present program was based on the principle that one approach cannot fit the needs and capacities of all people seeking treatment. A variety of methods and information compiled into a short-term package could begin to give people the tools with which to work to alleviate their depression. Goals for the group were to provide symptomatic relief (not symptom removal), to impart information, to identify problem areas that might be contributing to the patient's depression, and to begin developing coping skills to deal with these problems.

A sampling of patients who have benefited from the therapy experience described in this chapter includes an unemployed truck driver with an eighth grade education who lost his job after a back injury. Unable to secure employment, he lost his house and his second wife subsequently left him. He sought treatment after he began to have thoughts of suicide.

Another patient was a 35-year-old woman who was raped, who lost her job due to a life-threatening illness, and whose three school-age children were forced to live with their father because she could no longer provide for them. Although not suicidal, she presented with symptoms of anxiety and depression that impaired her capacity to manage on a daily basis.

Other patients presented with more long-standing difficulties, having battled recurrent bouts of depression, with histories of dysfunctional or abusive families and relationships, and limited coping capacities. It is clear that the clinical outcome of this therapy experience for these types of patients will not be as positive as that for patients with a more recent acute onset of difficulties. Selection criteria for any group should consider these variables.

Selection of members is crucial. However, there is some latitude in the definition of appropriate criteria. Some authors advocate exclusion if the patient is psychotic, has borderline personality disorder, or is self-destructive or violent (Budman and Bennett 1983). Others add inclusionary criteria of a more acute onset of difficulties, the ability to relate interpersonally with others, and the absence of extreme dependence or aggressiveness (Butcher and Koss 1978). Klein (1985) stated that many of the selection criteria put forth in the literature can be regarded by therapists in a typical outpatient clinic as "frivolously luxuriant" or "irrelevant" for the majority of patients referred for group therapy.

One study of referrals for group therapy in a large university hospital setting showed that the majority were for moderately to severely disturbed individuals, mostly single white women from middle- and working-class backgrounds, university students, or poorly educated, unemployed minority patients (Klein and Carroll 1986). It is Klein's opinion that "more seriously disturbed, chronically ill, or less well-motivated patients also can benefit from a short-term therapy group. However, if such patients are selected, then the goals of the group, its structural features, and the role and techniques of the therapist need to be tailored accordingly" (Klein 1985, p. 316).

Those patients not deemed appropriate for treatment with this particular group format were those who exhibited major psychotic/melancholic depression, schizophrenia in partial remission with depressive features, organic impairment, or borderline intelligence. Patients with character pathology such as borderline personality organization or antisocial or schizotypal personality characteristics have difficulty relating interpersonally and cannot make sufficient use of the cognitive material presented in this short-term group experience. Patients with a dual diagnosis, such as substance abuse and depression, are also difficult to treat with this model. Although some benefit is gained from the information and interaction of the group, the substance abuse issues must be dealt with through some other form of treatment if these patients are to receive any benefit from this therapy experience. The setting of appropriate goals for treatment in the group for each individual is most important because of the range of severity and chronicity of symptoms.

Group Composition and Member Preparation

Many authors writing from an interpersonal/psychodynamic theoretical orientation recommend heterogeneity of patient characteristics, symptoms, and problems. At the same time, homogeneity in regard to ego strength and capacity to tolerate anxiety is seen as desirable. Variety in personality and emotional problems is believed to prevent reinforcement of problems and to facilitate communication among members (Kaplan and Sadock 1993; Poey 1985; Yalom 1985). However, the recent literature on short-term groups supports the use of homogeneous groups organized around a focal problem or theme (Flowers and Booraem 1991; Klein 1985). In these kinds of groups, members share a sense of commonality that promotes the rapid development of cohesion. It is easier to feel closer to and less threatened by people who are perceived as having similar qualities. This sense of commonality or similarity also promotes other curative factors—for example, vicarious and interpersonal learning, acceptance, universality, and the instillation of hope—that have been cited as helpful in short-term therapeutic groups (Brabender et al. 1983; Maxmen 1973).

In the treatment program described in this chapter, group members all share depressive illness, either long-standing or of more acute onset. The members are more heterogeneous in regard to sex, race, and socioeconomic factors, with most falling between the ages of 30 and 50 and from lower- and middle-class backgrounds. It should be noted that studies point to the efficacy of brief, structured helping interventions with individuals from lower- and working-class backgrounds (Lorion 1974, 1978).

Present evidence supports the use of some form of pretherapy preparatory training (Garvin 1990; Piper and Perrault 1989; Poey 1985). Pretherapy training can correct patient misconceptions, and facilitate the development of appropriate group norms, which contribute to the ability of the group and individuals to work on goal attainment. Preparation of group members can be done individually, but some authors have found group training to be particularly helpful in preparing for group therapy (Budman and Bennett 1983; Rose 1989).

This model uses both individual and group pretherapy training sessions to prepare members for group participation. Individual interviews are found helpful with those individuals who express a high degree of concern or uncomfortable feelings about participating in a group. Rules and expectations of the group are explicitly stated at both individual and group pretherapy sessions to foster the development of therapeutic group norms. Potential members are given the opportunity to decide if they wish to participate in the group at the pretherapy training session and are asked to complete instrumentation that will help focus treatment and gauge therapeutic outcome.

Structure and Leadership

A study of short-term group therapy consisting of 16 sessions (Flowers and Booraem 1991) compared structured psychoeducational groups and less-structured, experiential groups whose members had heterogeneous psychological problems. Patients in the structured groups improved significantly more on the Automatic Thoughts Questionnaire (Kendall and Hollon 1994), a measure of overall pathology based on DSM-III, and on a target goals measure (Battle et al. 1966) than did patients in the experiential groups. The authors raise the possibility that it is structure in short-term therapeutic groups rather than homogeneity that contributes to therapeutic outcome. It seems logical to assume that groups are easier to structure if the members have similar problems, socioeconomic status, or other characteristics, such as stage in the adult developmental life cycle. Structured groups are also more effective than unstructured groups for divorce adjustment (Kessler 1978), psychiatric inpatients (Pekula et al. 1985), and problem solving (deAnda 1985).

The group leader can use activities and interventions to structure group interaction to aid the development of a meaningful and positive therapeutic learning environment. In a thoughtful discussion of leadership in short-term therapeutic groups, Dies (1985) stated that leaders must intervene actively to manage boundaries, maintain task focus, and regulate the intensity of emotional expression. These activities need not be manipulative and controlling of the group process, but rather are facilitative, and aid in the achievement of mutually agreed-on patient goals.

Lundgren (1979), in a study of T-group leadership, concluded that leaders play a significant role in facilitating an open and supportive atmosphere within the group. The group leader actively intervenes to foster supportive interactions and make connections of similarities among group members. The leader also lessens the possibilities for confrontational exchanges, especially early in the group's development and with members who have more severe pathology. Research on groups in laboratory and training settings has shown that positive feedback is almost always rated as more desirable, having greater impact, and leading to greater intention to change than negative feedback, and that behaviorally oriented feedback is more effective than emotional feedback (Dies 1985).

Bednar et al. (1974), after reviewing the literature, hypothesized that high levels of structure in the beginning stage of therapy would be beneficial to all group members: " . . . lack of structure in early sessions not only fails to facilitate early group development but actually feeds patient distortions, interpersonal fears, and subjective distress, which interfere with group development and contribute to premature patient dropout" (p. 36). Lower levels of patient responsibility for the conduct of the early group meetings allow members to engage in therapeutically relevant behaviors, such as self-disclosure and interpersonal feedback, more quickly and with less discomfort.

The introduction and sequencing of structure is also important. In a study designed to investigate the interaction of high and low degrees of leader structure and locus of control, Kinder and Kilmann (1976) found that high initial leader structure followed by a relatively unstructured leader role at the midpoint of treatment fostered greater gains in self-actualization than did other sequencings of structure. Other authors have also posited that such structure, tailored to the specific needs of the group, can help patients cope with the anxiety engendered by a new experience, and increase interpersonal functioning (Vitalo 1971; Weinstein and Pollack 1972). In a report on four studies of short-term group therapy, Flowers and Booraem (1989) demonstrated that when patients are specific about the problems or goals for therapy, disclose these problems in the group, and spend time discussing them with some reduction in emotional intensity, there tends to be therapeutic improvement.

Guided by this information, our group model was designed with a high degree of structure in the initial stages of the group through the use of structured exercises and leader interventions designed to both elicit and impart information and to promote the rapid development of cohesion among group members. As the group progresses through developmental stages, there is less structure of the sessions through the use of exercises and activities, although these tools continue to be used to some degree throughout the group process. Leader interventions become more directed to the facilitation of group interaction and problem solving and to the development of linkages between people.

Psychotherapy and Learning Styles

Learning theory has had a significant impact on both individual and group psychotherapy by elucidating mechanisms of learning and behavioral change (Bandura 1977a, 1977b). Lectures and exercises directed toward specific issues are what differentiates psychoeducational formats from traditional process groups. Information is purposefully imparted via a variety of experiences. Lessons address common concerns shared by group members along the chosen focus. Through the stages of group process and development, members progress from recognition of common concerns to a greater understanding and acceptance of their difficulties. With the use of proper material and exercises, members can move from experiencing to more risk taking and sharing in the group, which will lead to a larger range of behavioral choices in dealing with problem situations. It is most important to choose materials and build exercises that take into account the needs and capacities of the members, the overall goals of the group, and the phase of the treatment process (Ettin et al. 1988).

Although therapy is widely seen as a learning experience, the application of the theory of learning styles has received little attention in the literature, and then mainly in regard to the teaching of social skills to adults with severe psychiatric disability. Learning can be viewed as an interactive process involving both the teaching method employed and the style of the learner. "Learning style" has come to describe a specific subset of learner and contextual variables that directly affect both learning and teaching (Stawar 1992). Learning styles are characterized as a preference for using auditory or verbal, visual, tactile, or kinesthetic means for the acquisition of information and learning. Other contextual factors include time, space, light preference, and solitude (Dunn and Dunn 1978). Most individuals have a characteristic preference and predominantly use one means for acquiring information.

Although auditory or verbal learning is used mainly with adults, and therapy has been called "the talking cure," not all adults learn best through these means; sometimes a combination can better address the divergent needs of adults. Stawar's (1992) study of the learning styles of severely psychiatrically impaired adults pointed to the use of auditory means for the primary presentation of material and then reinforcement through visual, kinesthetic, and tactile modalities. Team learning and small-group techniques (e.g., case studies) can also be beneficial.

The use of visual, tactile, and kinesthetic methods of learning is most readily seen in creative arts therapies. There is a body of theoretical literature that suggests that the creative arts can induce therapeutic processes that aid patients in ways that are different from verbal therapies (Zwerling 1979). Other authors have stated that the use of art materials can bypass intellectual defenses by accessing emotions more directly, and that anxiety related to these feelings is reduced by the structure and symbolic representation inherent in such materials (Cardone et al. 1982; Robbins 1980). These kinds of activities shared in a group can contribute to the rapid development of cohesion in short-term therapy.

Application of this information in our model is seen in the use of mini-lectures and discussions, often followed by readings, the occasional use of writing assignments, and the use of collage materials and photographs. Although some members express initial reluctance to use these materials, most have found them to be very meaningful in expressing their difficulties, particularly the collage-making activity of Session 2. Group members are explicitly told that although verbal means are the primary vehicle used for therapeutic learning in the group, not all individuals respond best to this approach and a variety of means are therefore necessary to meet individual needs. Reading materials are provided for use between sessions, and brief written exercises are used both during and between sessions. Individual styles and differences are stressed and attempts are made to help group members feel successful in participating in the group through these different means.

Depression

Depression is probably one of the most universal of human problems. Although symptomatology varies somewhat as a function of culture and ethnicity (Levitt et al. 1983), in Western society it is estimated that between 10% and 20% of the population have symptoms severe enough to seek treatment (Lewinsohn et al. 1986; Regier et al. 1988). Depression is the most common problem reported by the elderly and is a growing problem for adolescents and children as well (Levitt et al. 1983). Several studies point to the fact that depression occurs in women at a ratio of 2:1 over men (Weissman and Klerman 1992).

Present classification systems recognize that depression can arise as a reaction to stressful life events or loss, or can be a long-standing difficulty as seen in dysthymia or chronic depression, with the possibility of a genetic predisposition. There does seem to be some relationship between less education, lesser income, and lower socioeconomic factors and increased depression (Levitt et al. 1983). Stressful life events can also play a role in depressive episodes. The increased likelihood of depression can be a reaction to coping with chronic stress, loss, and perceptions of failure (Wolman and Stricker 1990).

Group therapy is widely used in the treatment of nonmelancholic depression. Research results suggest that group interventions are effective in the alleviation of depressive symptoms with outpatient populations (Antonuccio et al. 1984; Lewinsohn et al. 1986; Marshall and Mazie 1987; Teri and Lewinsohn 1986; Vandervoort and Fuhriman 1991; Yost 1986). Most of the research done on group treatment of depression has involved cognitive or behavioral interventions; however, research on both individual and group treatment indicates that psychodynamic and interpersonal therapeutic strategies are also effective in the treatment of depression (Piper et al. 1992). There can be common factors that play an active role in all of these treatments (Lambert et al. 1986).

Translating Theory Into Practice: Structured Group Treatment of Depression

An intervention using the varied theoretical models of depression needs to impart information, such as the statistics and symptoms of depression; possible physical and emotional causes; some of the main theories about depression; the roles of cognitions, behaviors, stress, loss, and interpersonal relationships; and various possible coping strategies associated with the theories. Given the social nature of depression, the possible social etiologic factors, and the social effects of isolation and withdrawal, a group format for dealing with these issues is a most appropriate intervention. A group can provide the needed social support, reality testing, and feedback about behaviors that could mitigate against the debilitating effects of depression. The small group can be the treatment of choice for problems in interpersonal relationships and functioning (Northen 1988).

The appendix to this chapter provides an outline and discussion of each group session and illustrates how theoretical formulations are used to shape therapeutic endeavors. For each session, the relevant theory undergirding the format is reviewed. Specific goals are then presented and information is purposefully disseminated through the use of lectures and exercises. The structure of the sessions is designed to promote the move from recognition, understanding, and acceptance of information, to beginning application in the lives of group members.

Conclusions

In this chapter, I have described a time-limited, structured group program based on a variety of theoretical principles to provide treatment for depressed patients. Members are educated about the symptoms and possible causes of their symptoms, as well as about the various theories and rationales for understanding depression. Structured activities are used to facilitate the recognition and expression of feelings and cognitions associated with depression. Patients have an opportunity to practice instituting specific changes in their lives. The interpersonal context in which depression can develop is also explored.

Some limitations of this model can be identified. The breadth and scope of the material is considerable and can overwhelm some patients. The time limitation can lead to a lack of sufficient practice in applying various coping strategies and skills presented. Preliminary research results using the Beck Depression Inventory (Beck and Steer 1987) and the Symptom Checklist–90 (Derogatis 1977) show evidence of clinical efficacy. A major advantage of the model is that it is not likely to do harm to the participants.

Further research and refinement of this model will focus on what types of patients show the best clinical outcomes, what components are the most efficacious, and what is the optimum sequencing of the material. It is most important to remember that every group is unique, and that although this is a sensible model that can be defended theoretically, it is still a framework on which therapeutic work must be flexibly draped and rearranged to meet the needs of the individuals and the group.

The goal of developing a multimodal treatment program that is grounded in empirical research literature is ambitious. This protocol represents a systematic effort to create a time-limited format that can be applied in diverse service settings and with a broad range of clinical populations. It can be the only treatment offered, or can be used in conjunction with antidepressant medication, as detailed in the American Psychiatric Association Practice Guideline for Major Depressive Disorder in Adults (1993).

References

Abraham K: Selected Papers of Karl Abraham (1911). London, Hogarth Press, 1927

American Psychiatric Association: Practice guideline for major depressive disorder in adults. Am J Psychiatry 150 (suppl):1–26, 1993

Antonuccio D, Thompson A, Chatham P, et al: An exploratory study: the psycho-educational group treatment of drug-refractory unipolar depression. J Behav Ther Exp Psychiatry 15:309–313, 1984

Averill JR: Anger and Aggression: An Essay on Emotion. New York, Springer-Verlag, 1982

Bandura A: Social Learning Theory. Englewood Cliffs, NJ, Prentice-Hall, 1977a

Bandura A: Self-efficacy: toward a unifying theory of change. Psychol Rev 84:191–215, 1977b

Battle CC, Imber SD, Hoehn-Saric R, et al: Target complaints as criteria of improvement. Am J Psychother 20:184–192, 1966

Beck AT: Cognitive Therapy and the Emotional Disorders. New York, International Universities Press, 1976

Beck AT, Steer RA: Beck Depression Inventory Manual. New York, Harcourt Brace Jovanovich, 1987

Bednar RL, Melnick J, Kaul TJ: Risk, responsibility, and structure: a conceptual framework for initiating group counseling and psychotherapy. J Counsel Psychol 21:31–37, 1974

Benson H: The Relaxation Response. New York, William Morrow, 1975

Berne E: Transactional Analysis in Psychotherapy. New York, Grove, 1961

Brabender V, Albrecht E, Sillitti J, et al: A study of curative factors in short-term group psychotherapy. Hosp Community Psychiatry, 34:643–644, 1983

Budman SH, Bennett MJ: Short-term group psychotherapy, in Comprehensive Group Psychotherapy, 2nd Edition. Edited by Kaplan HI, Sadock BJ. Baltimore, MD, Williams & Wilkins, 1983, pp 138–144

Burns DD: The Feeling Good Handbook. New York, William Morrow, 1980

Butcher JN, Koss MP: Research on brief and crisis-oriented psychotherapies, in Handbook of Psychotherapy and Behavior Change, 2nd Edition. Edited by Bergin AE, Garfield SL. New York, Wiley, 1978, pp 725–767

Cardone I, Marengo J, Calisch A: Conjoint use of art and verbal techniques for the intensification of the therapeutic group experience. The Arts in Psychotherapy 9:263–268, 1982

deAnda D: Structured vs. nonstructured groups in the teaching of problem solving. Social Work in Education 7:80–89, 1985

Derogatis LR: SCL–90 Administration, Scoring and Procedures Manual: I. Baltimore, MD, Johns Hopkins University Press, 1977

Dies RR: Leadership in short-term therapy: manipulation or facilitation? Int J Group Psychother 35:435–455, 1985

Dunn R, Dunn K: Teaching Students Through Their Individual Learning Styles: A Practical Approach. Reston, VA, Reston Publishing, 1978

Ettin MF, Heiman M, Kopel SA: Group building: developing protocols for psychoeducational groups. Group 12:205–225, 1988

Ferster CB: A functional analysis of depression. Am Psychol 28:857–870, 1973

Flowers JV, Booraem CD: Four studies toward an empirical foundation for group therapy [Special issue: advances in group work research]. Journal of Social Service Research 13:105–121, 1989

Flowers JV, Booraem CD: A psychoeducational group for patients with heterogeneous problems: process and outcome. Small Group Research 22:258–273, 1991

Garvin CD: Short term group therapy, in Handbook of the Brief Psychotherapies. Edited by Wells RA, Gianetti VJ. New York, Plenum, 1990, pp 513–536

Gaylin W: The Rage Within: Anger in Modern Life. New York, Simon & Schuster, 1984

Harris TA: I'm O.K.—You're O.K.: A Practical Guide To Transactional Analysis. New York, Harper & Row, 1969

Holmes TH, Rahe RH: The social readjustment rating scale. J Psychosom Res 11:213–218, 1967

Jacobson E: Progressive Relaxation. Chicago, IL, University of Chicago Press, 1938

Kaplan HI, Sadock BJ: Structured interactional group psychotherapy, in Comprehensive Group Psychotherapy, 3rd Edition. Edited by Kaplan HI, Sadock BJ. Baltimore, MD, Williams & Wilkins, 1993, pp 324–338

Kendall PC, Hollon SD: Automatic thoughts questionnaire, in Measures for Clinical Practice: A Source Book, 2nd Edition. Edited by Fischer J, Corcoran K. New York, Free Press, 1994, p 71

Kessler S: Building skills in divorce adjustment groups. Journal of Divorce 2:209–216, 1978

Kinder BN, Kilmann PR: The impact of differential shifts in leader structure on the outcome of internal and external group participants. J Clin Psychol 32:857–863, 1976

Klein RH: Some principles of short-term group therapy. Int J Group Psychother 35:309–329, 1985

Klein RH, Carroll RA: Patient characteristics and attendance patterns in outpatient group psychotherapy. Int J Group Psychother 36:115–132, 1986

Klerman GL, Weissman MM, Rounsaville BJ, et al: Interpersonal Psychotherapy of Depression. New York, Basic Books, 1984

Lambert MJ, Shapiro DA, Bergin AE: The effectiveness of psychotherapy, in Handbook of Psychotherapy and Behavior Change, 3rd Edition. Edited by Garfield SL, Bergin AE. New York, Wiley, 1986, pp 157–211

LeCroy CW: Anger management or anger expression: which is most effective? Residential Treatment for Children and Youth 5:29–39, 1988

Levitt EE, Lubin B, Brooks JM: Depression: Concepts, Controversies, and Some New Facts, 2nd Edition. Hillsdale, NJ, Lawrence Erlbaum, 1983

Lewinsohn PM, Munoz RF, Youngren MA, et al: Control Your Depression. New York, Prentice Hall, 1986

Lorion RP: Patient and therapist variables in the treatment of low income patients. Psychol Bull 81:344–354, 1974

Lorion RP: Research on psychotherapy and behavior change with the disadvantaged, in Handbook of Psychotherapy and Behavior Change, 2nd Edition. Edited by Garfield SL, Bergin AE. New York, Wiley, 1978, pp 903–938

Lundgren DC: Authority and group formation. Journal of Applied Behavioral Science 15:330–345, 1979

Marshall TK, Mazie AS: A cognitive approach to treating depression. Social Casework 68:540–545, 1987

Maxmen JS: Group therapy as viewed by hospitalized patients. Arch Gen Psychiatry 28:404–408, 1973

Northen H: Social Work With Groups, 2nd Edition. New York, Columbia University Press, 1988

Novaco RW: The cognitive regulation of stress and anger, in Cognitive-Behavioral Interventions: Theory, Research, and Procedures. Edited by Kendall PC, Hollon SD. New York, Academic Press, 1979, pp 241–285

Pekula RJ, Siegel JM, Farrar DM: The problem solving support group: structured group therapy with psychiatric inpatients. Int J Group Psychother 35:391–409, 1985

Piper WE, Perrault EL: Pre-therapy preparation for group members. Int J Group Psychother 39:17–34, 1989

Piper WE, McCallum M, Azim HFA: Adaptation to Loss Through Short-Term Group Psychotherapy. New York, Guilford, 1992

Poey K: Guidelines for the practice of brief, dynamic group therapy. Int J Group Psychother 35:331–354, 1985

Regier DA, Boyd JH, Burke JD, et al: One-month prevalence of mental health disorders in the United States: based on five Epidemiologic Catchment Area sites. Arch Gen Psychiatry 45:977–986, 1988

Robbins A: Expressive Therapy: A Creative Arts Approach to Depth Oriented Treatment. New York, Human Sciences Press, 1980

Rose S: Working With Adults in Groups: Integrating Cognitive-Behavioral and Small Group Strategies. San Francisco, CA, Jossey-Bass, 1989

Seligman MEP: Helplessness: On Depression, Development and Death. San Francisco, CA, Freeman, 1975

Selye H: Stress Without Distress. New York, Harper & Row, 1974

Stawar TL: Learning styles of adults with severe psychiatric disability: implications for psychoeducational programming. Psychosocial Rehabilitation Journal 15:69–76, 1992

Teri L, Lewinsohn PM: Individual and group treatment of unipolar depression: comparison of treatment outcome and identification of predictors of successful treatment outcome. Behavior Therapy 17:215–228, 1986

Vandervoort DJ, Fuhriman A: The efficacy of group therapy for depression, a review of the literature. Small Group Research 22:320–338, 1991

Vitalo RL: Teaching improved interpersonal functioning as a preferred mode of treatment. J Consult Clin Psychol 35:166–171, 1971

Weinstein MS, Pollack HB: The use of exercises in sensitivity training: a survey. Comparative Group Studies 3:497–512, 1972

Weisinger H: Dr. Weisinger's Anger Work-Out Book. New York, Quill, 1985

Weissman MM, Klerman GL: Depression: current understanding and changing trends. Annu Rev Public Health 13:319–339, 1992

Wolman BB, Stricker G: Depressive Disorders: Facts, Theories, and Treatment Models. New York, Wiley, 1990

Yalom ID: The Theory and Practice of Group Psychotherapy, 3rd Edition. New York, Basic Books, 1985

Yost EB (ed): Group Cognitive Therapy: A Treatment Approach for Depressed Older Adults. New York, Pergamon, 1986

Zwerling I: The creative arts therapies as "real therapies." Hosp Comm Psychiatry 30:841–844, 1979

Appendix: Depression Group Outline

Session 1

Rationale

There have been numerous theories of depression over the years, each with its own way of explaining causal processes. These theories can be classified into four general categories: biological, behavioral, cognitive, and interpersonal. It is important for individuals with depression to have an understanding of these theories and how they relate to their own situations. Each of these views has something to add to our understanding of the complex phenomenon of depression. An overview of these theories is presented during the session, with group members encouraged to apply them to their own lives. In keeping with the findings of Bednar et al. (1974) and Kinder and Kilmann (1976), a high degree of structure by the leader is characteristic of this session. Group norms are reiterated and reinforced. Beginning anxiety of group members and the development of the goal of group cohesion are addressed through the use of the structured introductory activity (Ettin et al. 1988; Vitalo 1971; Weinstein and Pollack 1972). Moreover, the formation of individual goals, which has been found to be related to positive therapeutic outcome (Flowers and Booraem 1989), is begun with this activity.

Goals

1. To gain understanding of signs and symptoms of depression. To understand the difference between sadness and depression.
2. To recognize the theories of depression: social learning or behavioral, cognitive, psychodynamic, and interpersonal.
3. To meet with others and share common experiences to reduce isolation and give support.
4. To begin to clarify individual goals.

Session Format

I. Overview of Group and Content
Brief lecture format (approximately 10 minutes). Some of this material was covered in the pretherapy training session.

A. Goals of group.
B. Format, attendance, assignments, confidentiality.
C. Rationale and content.
D. Overview of coping strategies.

> 1. Knowledge and information as sources of power.
> 2. Sharing and problem solving with others.
> 3. Positive self-talk.
> 4. Relaxation and stress management skills.
> 5. Pleasant activities.
> 6. Positive communication and relationship skills.
> 7. Working out grief and anger.

II. Group Exercise
Introductions. This exercise takes up 30–45 minutes of the session because members are encouraged to "tell their stories," and the leader points out common themes. The goal is to build group cohesion and to begin to define individual goals. This is a structured group process exercise.

A. "Four Corners" index card; one word/phrase to describe:

> 1. You as a person.
> 2. You when you are depressed.
> 3. You when you are not depressed.
> 4. What you hope to gain from participation in the group (begin to work on individual goals).

III. Brief Lecture (approximately 20 minutes)

A. Statistics on depression in population.
B. Signs and symptoms.
C. Theories of depression (more detailed).

IV. Group Discussion
Group discussion is to promote cohesion, make linkages between members, and check understanding and relevance of material.

Alternate group activity (depending on group needs). A case study, which is a written example of the history and symptoms of a person with depression, can be used with groups whose members are more reticent about participation or groups that have more low-functioning members. The case study can be done in pairs, with partners sharing similarities and dissimilarities in a less-threatening manner than if done in the entire group.

V. Homework Assignment
Home recording chart of depression. Members are asked to rate their level of depression using a simple Likert-type scale of subjective distress over any 5-day period during the next week. This is to be done four times a day: before breakfast, lunch, dinner, and bedtime. They are encouraged to notice their patterns, and if they are related to stressful situations or events. They are also encouraged to notice those times when they feel less depressed. (These activities have a psychoeducational focus.)

Session 2

Rationale

Information and knowledge can empower individuals to deal with their difficulties more effectively. This session continues a high degree of structure using written and creative exercises and presents information didactically through lecture and handouts. This helps group members deal with anxiety and build cohesion (Vitalo 1971; Weinstein and Pollack 1972). The charting of depression levels and discussion of individual patterns in the experience of depressive events is important for individual goal setting. Physical and biological information about depression is presented briefly and outlined in a handout, with patients encouraged to ask questions and discuss the information with their physicians. The first part of the session is clearly psychoeducational in nature (Ettin et al. 1988), and the second part more process oriented.

Using the theoretical information on the therapeutic use of art materials (Zwerling 1979) and learning styles (Dunn and Dunn 1978; Stawar 1992), a collage-making activity is a major part of the session. It usually takes at least an hour for all members to make and share the meanings of their creations. This group process is aimed at increasing group cohesion and sharing in a supportive environment. Many members have found this a most meaningful exercise, enabling them to access and express feelings in a new way.

Goals

1. To understand physical causes of depression.
2. To understand emotional causes of depression.
3. To recognize dangers and benefits of depression.
4. To recognize depressive patterns and the roles of thoughts, feelings, and actions in patterns.
5. To develop visual pictures of depression and share these with the group (process to rapidly build group cohesion).

Session Format

I. Review Homework
Depression rating chart (approximately 15 minutes of discussion and sharing). This can be done in small groups or dyads, depending on needs and capacities of individual members. At the end, each group reports.

A. Review chart of depression levels, best day/worst day.
B. How often did you get depressed?
C. When was the worst time?
D. What did it feel like to you?
E. What were you thinking?
F. What stressful event, if any, set it off?

II. Brief Lecture (approximately 10 minutes)

A. Physical causes of depression.
    1. Chemical imbalance.
    2. Endocrine disorders.

    3. Infectious diseases.
    4. Eating or sleeping habits.
    5. Medications.
B. Emotional causes of depression.
    1. Emotion: energy in motion.
    2. Unresolved conflicts and issues.
       a. Unresolved anger and hurt.
       b. Unresolved grief and loss.
       c. Unresolved identity conflicts.
C. Dangers and benefits of depression.

III. Creative Art Activity
Participants create a picture of their depression using various art materials, and share their pictures with the group.

IV. Group Discussion
Integrate session material and check for understanding of personal situation of self and others.

V. Homework Assignment
Depression recognition. Members are asked to report on a specific instance when they felt depressed, and to notice the circumstances of the situation, what they did, and the thoughts they had about the situation. This is in preparation for the next session's cognitive base.

Session 3

Rationale

This session uses the theoretical information about the importance of cognitive patterns in the onset and maintenance of depressive states. Structure through the use of exercises and directive leader interventions is still high, as posited by Bednar et al. (1974) and Kinder and Kilmann (1976). Individual target goals are further delineated and refined using the information from the previous sessions so that group members are more likely to experience therapeutic improvement (Flowers and Booraem 1989).

The last 25 years have seen a growing emphasis on the cognitive and behavioral views of depression. The cognitive view of depression postulates that negative automatic thoughts mediate between experience and action, causing feelings and actions associated with depression. Building on the ideas of Albert Ellis concerning irrational beliefs, Beck (1976) identified patterns of dysfunctional or distorted thinking as being the cause of depression. He stated that depressed persons possessed a cognitive triad of 1) a negative view of the self, 2) a negative view of the world, and 3) a negative view of the future. Schema or patterns of thought develop as a result of early experiences, which lead to faulty information processing. Beck's theory is a view of intrapsychic functioning influenced by cognitions. These thinking patterns influence how a person manages day-to-day living and social relationships.

Treatment involves cognitive restructuring, or changing negative thinking patterns by replacing them with more realistic ones. Because feelings are caused by thoughts, negative feelings can be managed by changing an individual's thinking patterns. More positive "self-talk" will lead to more positive feelings and interactions with the social environment (Burns 1980). This approach has received much empirical validation and is clinically useful in treating depression in both individual and group settings.

Goals

1. To understand 10 kinds of twisted thinking or cognitive distortions.
2. To recognize and discuss personal cognitive distortions.
3. To discuss and formulate alternative positive thoughts.

Session Format

I. Review Homework
Depressive episode recognition (this can take 15 to 20 minutes, depending on the nature of the group).

II. Brief Lecture (approximately 15 minutes)
Ten kinds of twisted thinking are identified, with a handout given for reinforcement.

A. All-or-none thinking.
B. Overgeneralization.
C. Mental filter.
D. Discounting the positive.
E. Jumping to conclusions.
F. Magnification/minimization.
G. Emotional reasoning.
H. "Should" statements.
I. Labeling.
J. Personification and blame.

III. Group Discussion
Recognize personal distortions and identify alternative positive thoughts. Each person shares an example of distorted thinking and formulates an alternative positive thought. This is the real "heart" of the session, with group members encouraged to share and come up with alternatives for one another, and can take as much as 30 minutes of the session or more.

   Alternate group activity (depending on group and individual needs).   Brief scenarios on cognitive distortions. Group receives a list of examples of the 10 distortions to recognize and solve, and members share their findings (can be done in dyads). This activity can be used with groups whose members are less verbal or have more difficulty grasping the concepts given in the brief lecture, because specific examples are given of each type of distortion.

IV. Target Goals
Use cards from first session, and work in pairs if necessary. Members should have sufficient information about depression and their own personal patterns to more accurately identify a major target goal and refine their initial goals. The issue of termination and achievement of individual goals is specifically mentioned in this activity.

V. Homework Assignment
Self-defeating thoughts exercise. Members are given a handout to be read between sessions to reinforce positive self-talk.

Session 4

Rationale

This session builds on the information of the preceding sessions but also introduces new information that will be used in the following sessions when the degree of structure will be less. This session allows time for discussion of issues related to group formation, which—according to stage development theory—arise after the initial engagement phase.

The behavioral view of depression grew out of social learning theory, which characterizes depression as a series of behaviors that can be learned under the same conditions of reward and reinforcement as other behaviors. Charles Ferster (1973) was the first behaviorist to study the behavior of depressed individuals; he found that they experienced a lack of positive outcomes from their behavior or an abundance of negative outcomes. Ferster stated that depressed individuals lacked the appropriate social skills necessary to foster positive interactions with others, and developed a program of social skills training that covered such areas as communication skills, assertiveness skills, and relaxation and stress management.

The idea of managing physical tension and emotional anxiety is not a new one. In 1938 Edmund Jacobson, a Chicago physician, published the book *Progressive Relaxation,* which outlined a deep-muscle relaxation technique. In 1975 Herbert Benson, also a physician, published *The Relaxation Response,* in which he theorized that if the body had a stress response as defined by Selye (1974), the body also had an equal and opposite response, which he called the *relaxation response.* Because excessive or chronic stress is implicated as a possible factor contributing to depression (Wolman and Stricker 1990), teaching of stress management and relaxation strategies has merit as a coping strategy for depression.

Goals

1. To review and evaluate sessions thus far, and to address issues of group formation.
2. To identify symptoms of stress, focusing on the physical, emotional, mental, and relational areas.

3. To understand and experience how progressive muscle relaxation can decrease stress and symptoms of depression.

Session Format

I. Review Homework
Self-defeating thoughts exercise (approximately 10 minutes of discussion).

A. Personal distortions and affirmations.
    1. Ask how doing homework was: any difficulties?
    2. What about affirmations: any difficulties?

II. Group Discussion
Length of discussion varies; usually approximately 20 minutes.

A. Personal reactions to group thus far.
    1. Discuss any difficulties or questions.
    2. Ask what has been helpful? What do members think would be helpful?

III. Brief Lecture (approximately 10 to 15 minutes)
Introduction to stress management.

A. Stress reaction (handout).
B. Relationship of stress, role changes, and transitions to depression (incorporates interpersonal theory about the stress of role changes and transitions, the grief process as stress).

IV. Group Discussion

A. What are your personal stressors and how have you coped with them?
B. What do you get from stress, both positive and negative?
C. How have these events and your efforts to cope with them affected your feelings of depression?

V. Relaxation Exercise

A.   Physical stress cues.
B.   Progressive muscle relaxation; use relaxation tape if group agrees.

VI. Homework Assignment
Relaxation handouts.

Session 5

Rationale

This session is designed to integrate and review material from previous sessions and to apply these to individual situations. Structure is being reduced and interventions are focused more on improving group inter-action and problem solving.

Interpersonal theories of depression encompass what happens both within and between individuals. In recognition of the fact that research on depression has uncovered the interpersonal nature of many depressive episodes, with the loss of significant relationships through death, divorce, or conflict and the lack of social support and intimate, confiding relationships contributing to depression, a short-term treatment for depression called *interpersonal psychotherapy* was developed.

This approach is based on the ideas of Adolph Meyer and Harry Stack Sullivan, whose work emphasized the importance of psychoso-cial and environmental influences on depression (Weissman and Kler-man 1984). Treatment focuses on interpersonal relations as found in four general problem areas: 1) grief and loss reactions; 2) role disputes or role transitions; 3) interpersonal difficulties such as marital disputes or a lack of intimate personal relations; and 4) social skills deficits.

Goals

1.   To review thinking patterns and alternate responses.
2.   To examine personal life events that have contributed to depressive symptoms.
3.   To consider these life events in terms of the four major areas of

grief, interpersonal disputes, role transitions, and interpersonal deficits.
4. To enhance mutual sharing and support.

Session Format

I. Review Homework
Review questions about handouts from previous session.

II. Group Exercise
Discuss major life events; use Holmes and Rahe (1967) scale.

A. What life events have the most significance?
B. What were the thought patterns and stress areas associated with these events?
C. What are alternate views of these events?

III. Group Discussion
Time to integrate the last two sessions, and how these apply to each person.

IV. Relaxation Exercise
Relaxation and breathing exercises; possible visualization exercise if individual capacities and needs allow.

V. Homework Assignment
Life events handout.

Session 6

Rationale

This session is a continuation of the examination of theoretical material regarding depression and its successful treatment, particularly as outlined by Ferster (1973), Lewinsohn (1974), and Antonuccio et al. (1984). Lewinsohn et al. (1986) developed a program that addresses the behaviors of depressed individuals, and looks at the presence or absence of both pleasurable and nonpleasurable activities. Their approach suggested that depressed individuals have few pleasurable activities and behaviors and that increasing these would decrease the symptoms of depression. A program was developed for increasing positive interactions with people and the environment using modeling, role playing, feedback about behaviors, and reinforcement for positive behaviors.

Relaxation and stress management skills are important in managing stress, loss, and rejection. Social skills, such as those taught in assertiveness training, and communication skills are important in managing and negotiating human relationships. Both the behavioral and the cognitive approaches have received empirical validation and have proven effective in treating unipolar depression in both individual and group formats. Social skills training, challenging of negative thinking, and increasing pleasurable activities can all be carried out within a small group. The goal is to reinforce learning from previous sessions.

Goals

1. To review behavioral theory of depression.
2. To examine relationship between pleasant activities and depression.
3. To examine activities that are likely to be experienced as pleasant.
4. To reinforce individual differences and coping abilities.
5. To remind members of termination, as this is halfway mark in the group sessions.

Session Format

I. Review Week and Homework (approximately 15 minutes)

A. Review how participants are handling feelings of depression.
B. Examine life changes that have contributed to depression.

II. Brief Lecture (approximately 10 minutes)

A. Review behavioral theory of depression.
B. Review relationship between pleasant activities and depression.
C. Examine activities likely to be experienced as pleasant.

III. Group Activity
Use pleasant activities scale.

A. Identify three pleasant activities and measure level of depression before, during, and after each activity.
B. Chart activity and share with group.

IV. Group Discussion
Each person chooses a favorite activity and shares it with the group. This activity and discussion take up the bulk of this group session.

A. What is different about the times when you are involved in a favorite or pleasant activity?
B. What would you do differently at these times?
C. What relationships and activities do you see as most important to your well-being?

V. Homework Assignment
Pleasant activities scale. Members are given two handouts on pleasant and social activities and are encouraged to engage in at least one pleasurable or social activity during the week and report back to the group about the experience.

Session 7

Rationale

Specific behaviors of individuals are more easily examined in a cooperative and positive atmosphere. Using the theoretical and empirical information on leadership (Dies 1985; Lundgren 1979) and feedback in groups (Dies 1985), the group structure has sought to foster such an atmosphere so that members engage in sufficient disclosure of problems, attitudes, and behaviors that contribute to depression.

This session reviews previous information and theory, particularly the social skills emphasis noted in the behavioral theoretical models (Ferster 1973; Lewinsohn et al. 1986), and also examines individual communication and social skills that are presented as work in the group session. This shift into the participants' own specific patterns, behaviors, and ways of relating to others is accomplished by reviewing the homework on pleasant and social activities and presenting a brief lecture on social and communication skills. The group discussion is focused on identifying characteristic patterns members have noticed in themselves and each other. Group members are encouraged to explore alternative ways of communicating and of handling problematic situations.

Goals

1. To review cognitive distortions and thinking patterns.
2. To further delineate pleasant activities and encourage action.
3. To explore social and communication skills and individual patterns.

Session Format

I. Review Homework
Pleasant activities scale (approximately 15 minutes).

A. What will have to happen for you to do more pleasant activities?
B. What activities do you need to do more?
C. What have you learned about yourself from this exercise?

II. Brief Lecture (approximately 15 minutes)
Focus on social and communication skills.

A. Meeting people, body language, eye contact.
B. Positive communication skills, "I" messages, assertiveness.

III. Group Discussion
Discuss communication styles and examine personal patterns (this takes up the bulk of the session).

A. What are problematic ways of communicating for each person?
B. What are problem situations and with whom do they occur?
C. What are alternative ways of communicating and handling these situations?

IV. Homework Assignment

Have group members do one pleasant activity and report back to the group. Pick one opportunity to do something different in a problem situation and report back to the group.

Session 8

Rationale

Group stage development theory specifies that sufficient cohesion should be established at this point in a group's development to allow for the examination of more personal information and issues. Examination of familial issues, negative emotionality, and their contribution to depressive symptoms is the theme in the next several sessions. Psychodynamic and interpersonal formulations of depression are reviewed. The degree of structure is further reduced in these sessions, shifting more of the locus of control from the leader to the group.

Early traumatic experiences, perceived losses, and impaired early relationships leave deficits in self-esteem and vulnerability to depression. Issues of unresolved grief and loss, and the underlying conflicts that accompany these, have been addressed in a psychodynamically oriented short-term group treatment program instituted at a large university hospital (Piper et al. 1992). A controlled clinical research evaluation of the treatment program revealed a strong treatment effect both statistically and clinically.

To make the psychodynamic theoretical material more accessible to group members, the colloquial terminology of ego states developed by Berne in transactional analysis (1961), and further popularized by Harris (1969), is used: parent, adult, and child. A handout is given that discusses the ego states and how each has a critical and nurturing aspect to it. The importance of the family in meeting early developmental needs for love and acceptance, and as early role models for learning interpersonal behaviors, is stressed in the brief lecture and the handout.

The homework assignment to bring in childhood family pictures is a relatively nonthreatening way to gain access to possibly painful material and issues of grief and loss, and also furthers group support and sharing of these issues. It allows for some creativity by group members, as indicated by a recent group member's compiling a videotape of her life, using old albums and clips of family reunions and activities. Many members find that they have few pictures of their childhood and some are motivated to seek out family sources for pictures. If pictures are not found, the painful experiences that lie behind this lack can be addressed.

Goals

1. To introduce dynamic theory using parent/adult/child approach.
2. To examine the impact of family and individual roles, and their contribution to present depressive symptoms.
3. To reinforce pleasant activities and positive communication.

Session Format

I. Review Homework
Review pleasurable activity and problem situation (approximately 15 minutes).

II. Brief Lecture (approximately 15 minutes)
Discuss dynamic model and parent/adult/child handout.

III. Group Activity
Self-esteem and family perceptions. This is a handout activity to be done in the group that addresses issues of how each member perceived their family and how they think others perceived their family. This activity and the ensuing discussion make up the bulk of this session.

A. Share perceptions with group.
B. Discuss the role your family played in your present depressive behaviors.

IV. Group Discussion
Discuss issues of unresolved grief, role changes in present family, and how family-of-origin issues affect present relationships and ways of communicating. Interpersonal theory can also be addressed again here for reinforcement.

V. Homework Assignment
Ask group members to bring childhood pictures to share at next meeting.

Session 9

Rationale

The group now has reached a developmental stage where work on relatively threatening interpersonal and negative emotional issues can take place. Interpersonal theory (Weissman and Klerman 1990), particularly in relation to problematic interpersonal relationships and issues of unresolved grief and loss, are reviewed along with other family-of-origin issues, such as unmet needs and ways of learning to cope with difficulties.

Goals

1. To further examine role of family in depression.
2. To review interpersonal theory, skill deficits, and how relationships affect depression.
3. To deepen sharing and help of the group.

Session Format

I. Review Week (approximately 10 minutes)
Determine how group members are doing with depression and individual goals. Individual goal sheets are reviewed and goal attainment is related to termination issues.

II. Group Sharing
Group members share pictures of childhood. This can take as much of the session as necessary to adequately address all issues.

A. Describe self and situation in picture.
B. What role did you play in your family?
C. How did you feel?
D. What connection do your past childhood experiences have with your present depression?

III. Brief Lecture
Review of interpersonal theory (can be omitted if discussion is going well).

A. How do present interpersonal relationships contribute to your present feelings of depression?
B. What is your part in these relationships?
C. What changes might improve these relationships?

IV. Group Discussion
Integrate material from session and discuss progress on personal goals.

Session 10

Rationale

The first person to postulate a relationship between anger and depression was psychoanalyst Karl Abraham (1927). Since that time, numerous studies have attempted to link repressed anger or internalized rage to clinical symptoms such as depression. Anger and the expression of anger can be very threatening to patients, with the fear being that the power of the anger will antagonize or alienate loved ones or others, and in the process harm or even destroy the person expressing the anger.

The psychodynamic theory of depression is understood by many authors as a manifestation of anger directed inward against the self rather than outward at the target of one's anger (Averill 1982). Other theorists such as Beck (1976), Lewinsohn (1974), and Seligman (1975) do not give any specific role to anger in the etiology of depression. Clinicians now delineate anger from aggression and see it as a factor in many illnesses, including depression. There is a peculiar relationship between anger and depression, because many depressed individuals fail to express anger, and in numerous reported cases the recognition and expression of anger has been a successful component of therapeutic relief (Gaylin 1984).

Other authors have proposed that the management and regulation of anger, or anger control through assertiveness training, is more effective than the mere recognition and expression of anger (LeCroy 1988; Novaco 1979; Weisinger 1985). Sessions 10 and 11 attempt to help group members identify, express, and find alternative ways of handling their present anger and of resolving past hurts.

Goals

1. To recognize signs of past anger.
2. To acknowledge hurt feelings.
3. To explore healthy ways of expressing anger, and more positive communication patterns.
4. To discuss termination issues related to anger and loss of the group.

Session Format

I. Review Week (approximately 10 minutes)
How are group members doing with feelings of depression; what's better? Begin to focus on gains and how group members are coping more positively; focus on maintenance of change.

II. Brief Lecture (approximately 10 minutes)
Discuss handout on anger.

A. Signs of anger.
B. Fears of expressing anger.
C. Recognizing past hurts.
D. Recognizing difficulties people have with endings—how issues of past losses, hurt, and anger can be reactivated.

III. Group Activity
Take Action (anger workout). This activity and discussion take up the bulk of the session.

A. List any symptoms that can reflect past anger.
B. Complete the following sentence:
   "I felt hurt when _____
   _____ and I am still hurting."
C. Write down what prevented you from expressing yourself.

IV. Group Discussion
Discuss personal signs of anger, situations that arouse angry feelings, and individual ways of handling anger.

V. Homework Assignment
Ask participants to write down one situation during the week in which they become angry, either in a close relationship or another situation, and bring it to the next group meeting.

Session 11

Rationale

Although termination has been an issue in treatment all along, with periodic reminders of the finite nature of the group, the final two sessions of the group are focused more on termination issues and the feelings aroused by the ending of the group. Possible feelings of abandonment, of not getting enough, or of feeling "pushed out" by an uncaring system are explored in the group and alternative ways of framing these feelings are actively explored.

Goals

1.   To continue to focus on positive communication skills.
2.   To identify and practice alternative ways of handling anger.
3.   To explore ways of increasing social contact and support.
4.   To address termination issues.

Session Format

I. Review Homework
Review group members' anger-producing situations.

A.   Describe situation—what you thought and did.
B.   Explore alternative ways of handling situation.
C.   What are some helpful ways you have discovered to express or handle anger?

II. Group Activity
Write a letter to someone with whom you have been angry. Share it with the group and discuss your feelings.

III. Group Discussion
Integrate session material, and discuss feelings about the group ending.

IV. Homework Assignment
Write a short sentence about a positive change you have made during group therapy, and bring it to the last session.

Alternate homework assignment. Write a short sentence for each person on separate pieces of paper about one positive change you have seen them make during the course of the group's meeting. Use this activity depending on level of cohesion in the group and functioning of individual members.

Session 12

Rationale

Material is reviewed through group discussion. Individual goals are reviewed and evaluated. Positive change is highlighted and strategies for maintaining change are explored. A personal and group evaluation of the experience is encouraged, with both strengths and weaknesses included. A positive termination experience is stressed by recognizing both the gains members have made and the issues that still need work.

Goals

1. To evaluate the personal and group aspects of the therapy experience.
2. To review goal attainment.
3. To create a positive termination atmosphere.

Session Format

I. Group Discussion

A.   What changes do you see in yourself since the group started?
B.   What have you learned and accomplished?
C.   How can you maintain your gains?
D.   What are your feelings about the group ending?

II. Group Activity

Group members share positive changes. Members are asked to complete any clinical research materials after the group is finished.

A.   Each member shares his or her positive changes and tapes them to a poster or wall.
B.   The leader participates in this activity by talking about the changes he or she sees in each member.
C.   Individual goals are reviewed.

Alternate group activity.   Members share what they have written about each person and give them the piece of paper.

Chapter 5

The Intensive Psychotherapy Center in the Managed Care Environment

Gerald C. Peterson, M.D.

*T*he intensive psychotherapy center (IPC) is part of a diverse set of clinical programs under the umbrella of the Department of Psychiatry and Psychology at the Mayo Clinic in Rochester, Minnesota. It is an intensive multimodal group therapy program that originated from a need to provide a setting for concentrated psychotherapy for general medical/surgical patients with a wide variety of problems. In this chapter, I review the historical development of the program, with a particular emphasis on the need to respond to the changing requirements of our patients as well as to pressures from the managed care environment.

Even though service programs such as ours have demonstrated the effectiveness of this style of group psychotherapy, external pressures have had an increasing impact on what we can provide to our patients. Case managers will ultimately decide who is eligible for these programs and for what duration of treatment. Consequently, service programs need to constantly reassess the role they are playing in the overall care of the patient and adapt to these outside pressures. We recently reviewed the mission and goals of our program in order to develop a new plan of action to help us adapt to managed care, as well as a move to a new clinical setting.

The IPC Program

The IPC program currently offers a core 3-week program that remains the heart of our activities. Even though it is an outpatient program, the patients participate on a full-time basis 7 hours a day, 5 days a week, with most patients staying for 3 weeks. In addition, the program provides less-intensive, long-term group therapy, individual psychotherapy, marital therapy, and individual psychiatric assessment. We have been fortunate to have a comfortable, relatively nonclinical setting for our activities in a large home located midway between our major inpatient and outpatient settings.

When the program began, the patient population came from a large catchment area in the Midwest. Many of these patients arranged to remain in Rochester for an intensive period of outpatient treatment. The context of a large general medical clinic resulted in a major proportion of patients with somatoform disorders as well as physical symptoms related to depression and anxiety. In recent years, however, a greater proportion of our patients identify interpersonal conflict and relationship issues as their primary reasons for attending the IPC program. The program is staffed by a psychiatrist who acts as consultant and supervisor. The groups are conducted by residents in psychiatry and/or by cotherapists who have masters-level degrees in nursing, social work, or psychology. The cotherapists have extensive experience in group therapy and play an active role in educating our psychiatry residents, who usually spend one quarter at the IPC.

Our overall goal is to provide a setting of confrontation with considerable support. Therapy approaches are varied and include group psychotherapy, individual therapy, psychodrama and sociograms, and facilitated video replay with a replay therapist. As shown in the schedule (Table 5–1), the patients spend a very busy day moving from one situation to another.

Although the modes of therapy used in our program are well known, their combination is rather unusual. This combination did not develop from any particular theoretical bias but rather evolved on a very pragmatic basis—whatever worked was used and continued. The various therapeutic settings promote the rapid exposure of maladaptive behavior patterns. This is a striking difference from long-term individual psychotherapy. The treatment modalities are complementary and highly integrated, allowing the patient to deal with the same issues from a number of perspectives. Issues that emerge overtly in one setting, such as psychodrama, may quickly become a focus in a core group psychotherapy hour. Themes and behaviors exhibited during a core psychotherapy group are immediately discussed in an objective manner

Table 5–1. Daily schedule of intensive psychotherapy center

8:00–9:00 A.M.	Staff conference; new patient introduction
9:00–10:00 A.M.	Core group psychotherapy
10:00–11:00 A.M.	Facilitated video replay; individual therapy
11:00 A.M.–12:00 P.M.	Psychodrama; sociograms
12:00–1:00 P.M.	Lunch together
1:00–2:00 P.M.	Core group psychotherapy
2:00–3:00 P.M.	Informal group; individual sessions
3:00–3:30 P.M.	Closing summary group
3:30 P.M.	Staff conference

during a video replay facilitated by a replay therapist other than the usual group cotherapist.

Historical Review

MacKenzie and Pilling (1972) published an article in the *International Journal of Group Psychotherapy* over 20 years ago describing the initiation of this program, which we consider a "granddaddy" of short-term intensive group therapy programs. Loren Pilling and Hal Martin, who were members of the psychiatry staff at the Mayo Clinic at that time, saw a need for development of an outpatient day clinic program to provide intensive psychiatric services for patients who lived outside of Rochester and were able to remain until their medical treatment was completed. Initially, psychotherapy was attempted through daily individual sessions while the patient was completing a medical examination at the Mayo Clinic. This was helpful, but the need for a more intensive, time-limited treatment program became progressively more obvious. Even though the prevailing wisdom at the time suggested that "real" psychotherapy had to occur over a long period of time, later outcome studies indicated that an intensive program of this sort could provide substantial sustained improvement.

Day treatment programs existing in other institutions were reviewed but found to be largely designed for patients with much more severe psychiatric illnesses. At that time, the concept of the intensive group therapy treatment was unique and no similar program had been described in the literature. A program was designed for intensive short-term treatment of patients with what were then described as neurotic or psychosomatic disorders, or both. Originally, it was housed in a renovated section of an older hospital building and was staffed by three psychiatry residents, a staff consultant, a registered nurse, a practical nurse with psychiatric experience, and an activities director.

The program included 1-hour core group psychotherapy experiences in the morning and again in the afternoon, a 2-hour session of occupational therapy consisting of arts and crafts activities, individual sessions of psychotherapy with a psychiatry resident, and a large summary group meeting for 45 minutes in the afternoon. These patient activities were bounded by meetings of the staff the first thing in the morning and the last thing in the afternoon. The originators of the program, by their own admission, were not sure that what they were doing would be effective.

MacKenzie and Pilling (1972) reviewed the first 100 patients who attended the program. The average age of the patients was 40 years and the average length of stay was 2 weeks. The distribution of diagnoses, using the then-current DSM-II terminology (American Psychiatric Association 1968), indicated that more than 42% had depressive symptoms and 34% had somatoform symptoms. Compared with patients seen today, problems in interpersonal relationships (particularly adjustment disorders) seem to be underrepresented. This finding was perhaps influenced by the diagnostic classification used at that time. The change measures battery consisted of psychiatric symptoms, interpersonal relationships, and overall functioning. Evaluations were conducted at admission, discharge, and at a 6-month follow-up contact.

Of the 69 patients rated as improved at the time of discharge, follow-up ratings were received from 52 patients, and 85% of these indicated they had maintained their improvement 6 months later. Thirty-one patients had been rated as not improved at the time of discharge. Twenty of these patients had attended the day treatment clinic for less than 1 week and an additional four had a psychotic illness or chronic alcoholism. The initial study also showed that 22 of 29 patients with somatoform symptoms who stayed for the entire program showed significant improvement. Patients with psychotic illness and alcoholism had the least satisfactory outcomes.

Swenson and Martin (1976) conducted a second outcome study a few years later. Patient questionnaires were given at admission, discharge, and at follow-up 8 months later. These consisted of the Minnesota Multiphasic Personality Inventory (MMPI; Hathaway and McKinley 1943), self-ratings of severity of disability, and self-reports of the primary symptoms identified at the time of admission. The MMPI data indicated significant overall improvement at the time of discharge and maintenance of the improvement at 8-month follow-up (Figure 5–1). Similarly, self-ratings of primary symptoms at discharge and at 8-month follow-up demonstrated sustained improvement in approximately 80% of patients (Figure 5–2). These improvement figures are compatible with more recent surveys of group psychotherapy outcome (Orlinsky and Howard 1986; Robinson et al. 1990; Smith et al. 1980).

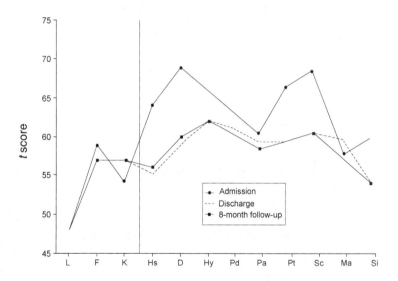

Figure 5–1. Mean patient scores on Minnesota Multiphasic Personality Inventory (MMPI; Hathaway and McKinley 1943) ($n = 140$). L = Lie Scale, F = Frequency Scale, K = Correction Scale, Hs = Hypochondriasis Scale, D = Depression Scale, Hy = Hysteria Scale, Pd = Psychopathic Deviance Scale, Pa = Paranoia Scale, Pt = Psychasthenia Scale, Sc = Schizophrenia Scale, Ma = Mania Scale, Si = Social Introversion Scale.

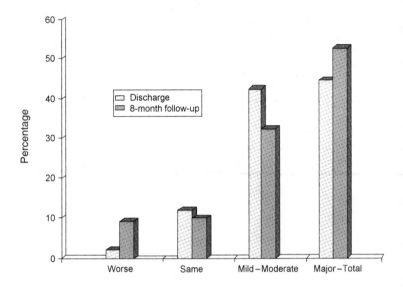

Figure 5–2.   Mean patient global improvement scores ($n = 140$).

It is interesting to review the changes in diagnostic composition over a 20-year period. The most recent data indicate that less than half as many patients now present with somatic symptoms as a primary concern, compared with the original study by MacKenzie and Pilling (1972). Three times as many patients present with interpersonal issues than in earlier periods (Table 5–2). This reversal is thought to be primarily reflective of a change in our referral base. In past years, most referrals were directly from the pool of general medical patients being assessed at the Mayo Clinic. Today, patients who have been assessed medically and determined to have somatoform disorder as a predominating symptom often either have access to adequate psychiatric help in their home communities or find that their health care plans require an initial treatment approach near their home communities. Currently, the greatest proportion of our referrals are from employee assistance programs and outpatient therapists serving the local population. Patients in this population are most often experiencing difficulty because of interpersonal and/or marital problems.

We have had no doubts about the efficacy of group therapy tech-

Table 5–2. Presenting symptoms on admission to the Intensive Psychotherapy Center

Symptom	MacKenzie 1972 (*n* = 100)	Swenson/Martin 1976 (*n* = 315)	Current 1991/1992 (*n* = 841)
Depression/dysphoria	42%	43%	35%
Somatic	34%	29%	14%
Interpersonal	None	11%	33%
Other	24%	17%	18%

niques in treating people manifesting depression, anxiety, and interpersonal problems. Because of the nature of our close alliance with the general medical and surgical services, we felt especially challenged to treat patients presenting predominantly with somatic symptoms and a diagnosis of somatoform disorder. We were pleased to find that the group of patients with somatoform disorders could be dealt with effectively and indeed had some of the best outcomes. Patients with somatoform disorders are particularly difficult to deal with because of their persistence in discussing somatic symptoms and their lack of psychological insight. Their transference to the therapist is of a dependent nature, seeking answers for their medical problems and wanting a direct explanation of their symptoms. In the intensive group format, this transference can be confronted rapidly and effectively, and the common negative reaction of the therapist toward these patients can be diluted. The multimodal approach allows observations of the waxing and waning of the patient's symptoms at times of heightened emotional expression in the group. By sharing mutual experiences with other patients with somatoform disorder, they are able to develop an increased sense of cohesion and feelings of mutuality, and are therefore able to increase their risk taking in group therapy sessions. A case vignette may illustrate how a patient with somatoform disorder responds to this treatment environment.

A 47-year-old single man was referred to the psychotherapy program by a psychiatrist who had evaluated him in consultation with the internist conducting his general medical examination. His symptoms included fatigue, weakness, gastrointestinal pain, a 35-pound weight loss, inability to continue his occupation for a month prior to his assessment, and feelings of depression. He had developed a fear of having cancer in the previous 6 months. The internist noted an inordinate preoccupation and concern with physical symptoms and diagnosed him as having depressive disorder and hypochondriacal disorder.

During the first week at the IPC, the patient continued to have a marked somatic focus, repeatedly expressing a fear of having cancer. He showed a good deal of anxiety in the group and had difficulty investing in the group process. However, during that first week he was also able to identify major concerns about his own aging, his elderly parents, and his loneliness. The group was able to point out his continuing dependency on his parents and during a psychodrama session his fear of vulnerability and denial of hostility became evident. He was able to review the videotape of the psychodrama session with feedback, allowing him to recognize these issues.

In the second week there was a decrease of somatic focus. The patient began to share his concerns about his sexuality with the therapist in an individual session after his group therapy session. He was able to return to the group to express these same concerns with affective sharing of shame and guilt. This was accepted by the group with a good deal of support. In the third week, he showed improved mood and was sleeping better. His somatic symptoms had decreased considerably. He was socializing more actively and showing more comfort with the other group members. He identified an attraction to a female group member.

Before dismissal the patient was able to recognize that his pain was experienced as symbolic punishment for intense guilt feelings about a past homosexual experience. He described a powerful corrective emotional experience in the group setting as he worked through feelings of shame and guilt and accepted validation by others, particularly by a female member of the group, of his attractiveness and value to others. At the time of dismissal his somatization had decreased dramatically. His depression was much less, and he developed significant psychological insight, being able to correlate his pain with emotional issues.

The resistance typical of somatizing patients can be reduced by treating them in a group with other patients who are more psychologically insightful or who have syndromes that are more readily identifiable as being emotionally related. By refocusing on behavioral and emotional issues, we hope to reduce the medical costs and need for hospitalization of our patients. These results have been demonstrated in other group therapy programs similar to ours (Weiner 1992).

Family members, usually the spouse, are strongly encouraged to participate in the program for at least 1 week during the 3-week stay. This participation facilitates identification of family behaviors that might be perpetuating the patient's pathology. The patient and family member can experience appropriate modeling of emotional—rather than somatic—expression of distress. They can objectively note pathological patterns through discussion and video replay, and can test out appropriate responses in the safety of the group setting. Inclusion of a spouse avoids discussions of conflict situations "outside" of the group setting itself. Interactions between the spouses can be observed in a valid way and pointed out immediately, thereby encouraging direct examination of the reality of the interactions and avoiding the common situation in which distorted views of a partner are expressed only when that person is absent.

Program Evolution

Outcome studies and clinical experience have shown our program to be highly effective for a variety of problems. Our goals have expanded over the past 25 years beyond symptom relief to increased self-knowledge and the development of higher-level coping skills. Various components have been added to complement the primary emphasis on small group psychotherapy.

Video Replay

We are impressed by the value of facilitated video replay. This technique was introduced at a relatively early point in the program's development and has been refined over the years. The video replay session is conducted by a therapist other than the primary cotherapist, and is scheduled with the core group immediately after a group session. Reviewing the group interactions on videotape allows the replay therapist to provide an objective view of the group process and avoids transference distortions by the group members. This objectification and opportunity to highlight important issues is found to facilitate the group process and also serves to educate patients to become more effective participant-observers of group function.

Psychodrama and Sociograms

Twice-weekly psychodrama and sociogram sessions are participated in by core group members. These sessions are planned by the therapist and structured in a way that brings out observed pathological interactions. This provides another way to overcome roadblocks in the therapeutic process.

Alcohol and Drug Abuse

An alcoholism counselor is present for one-half day per week. This was introduced because of the pervasive presence of substance abuse problems. Alcohol abuse and overt alcoholism is frequently a significant contributor to interpersonal and marital problems. At any point in time, 20%–30% of our patients show indications of alcohol or drug problems. These problems are addressed with the help of the alcoholism counselor, who meets individually with patients identified by their group cotherapist as having problems in this area.

Roles of Staff Clinicians

In addition to leading the groups, the masters-degree-level cotherapists now play a more direct role in diagnostic evaluation of individuals and couples. They also are more involved in the ongoing primary care of patients under the supervision of consulting psychiatrists. These roles have expanded rapidly as more efficient modes of delivering psychiatric care are explored. Having the therapists in the same facility as the supervising psychiatrist provides an effective forum for direct supervision.

Staff Burnout

Many of the patients now being seen for the group therapy program are those whose symptoms failed to respond to medications or short-term individual therapy. This is a direct result of the general practice of attempting brief crisis management or medications before referring patients to the IPC program. The intensive group psychotherapy experience has been found to be an excellent adjunct to individual therapy or psychopharmacological therapy. It allows the patient an opportunity to examine interpersonal interactions, conflicts, and pathological defenses not otherwise observable in individual counseling.

However, the intensity of the program extracts a great deal from the professionals who staff it. An additional reason for considering changes in the near future was to prevent staff burnout and to provide a greater variety of experiences in which they could use their considerable therapeutic skills. The therapists worked either in the core group program or with long-term groups for 1- or 2-year assignments. The psychological fatigue produced by long assignments is reduced by frequent supervision sessions and debriefings.

Even under the best of circumstances, burnout symptoms of negativism or cynicism can arise and be subtly destructive to the group process. Consequently, we plan to change the duration of assignments to 3- to 6-month intervals and will add a third assignment. In this third assignment, the therapist will interface with the entire outpatient program and have a variety of functions: individual therapist, consultant to employee assistance programs, cotherapist for a crisis intervention group, and evaluator of direct outpatient referrals.

Accommodations for the Program

The move from a hospital environment to the more comfortable nonclinical building in the early 1970s provided a more private setting in which to treat a growing local population of patients; it also contributed to a comfortable and educationally oriented milieu. Recently, the need for major renovations of the building, to meet current building codes, was encountered. In addition, there was the perception that the program needed better integration with overall outpatient services. Recognition of these needs resulted in a proposal to move to an outpatient clinical area, geographically closer to the outpatient psychiatric services.

Although the reasons for this move are understandable, there is uncertainty about the consequences of leaving the private, almost retreat-like, atmosphere of the present premises. The maintenance of an intensive milieu atmosphere is a key part of the program and a clear sense of spatial boundary is helpful for this to occur.

Changing Referral Patterns

Looking back over 25 years, it is apparent that we have not always adjusted promptly to external changes. When the IPC was first initiated, it was easy to refer patients into the program when it was obvious that they would benefit. Our outcome studies indicated that the program was useful and it could be easily justified to the patients. In the early years of the program, there was often a lack of effective psychiatric services for patients at home. Many of our patients came from smaller communities in the Midwest or other areas of the United States, and to receive psychiatric therapy required travel to large cities.

By contrast, most of the patients coming for medical consultation today have already consulted a psychiatrist, even for somatoform disorders, because access to effective psychiatric evaluation and care is available in smaller communities. We have seen our psychiatry residents develop group therapy skills and an enthusiasm for this form of therapy, which they have carried with them to establish programs of their own throughout the United States. We have also trained many group therapy cotherapists at our center. We seem to have created our own competition, certainly to the benefit of our patients but resulting in less need for patients to stay in the Rochester area to receive comparable care. Consequently, over the past two decades a greater proportion of patients have come from the local community. Currently, only 10% of patients are from outside the Midwest and half are from the city of Rochester itself.

A majority of patients referred to the program are women. Over the time the program has operated, a large number of women have begun pursuing careers or are in job situations that make it difficult for them to break away for a 3-week period of intensive psychotherapy. Even locally, managers and supervisors are encouraging their employees to seek psychotherapy in a way that will interfere minimally with their full-time job requirements, preferring their employees to be away from the job situation less frequently or to seek therapy during evening hours after work.

Insurance carriers now require a complex precertification process before they permit their patients to participate in our program. We developed patient brochures and papers of explanation that are provided to insurance carriers, and they have been reasonably supportive in allowing patients to participate for 3 weeks. Nevertheless, the required obstacles interfere with a smooth referral process. Some requirements, such as a need to update the patient's mental status exam weekly, seem inappropriate for our patients and indicate a lack of real understanding of the program by the insurance carriers.

The effectiveness of antidepressants for patients with somatoform and depressive disorders, combined with supportive psychotherapy, has been established. Physicians, their patients, and indeed the third-party payers may prefer this approach initially before participation in a more intensive psychotherapeutic intervention. This may be cost effective, but it does steer a large group of patients away from an intensive therapeutic program.

As a result of these changes, it has become apparent that there is a reduced requirement for the intensive program. Consequently, we have cut back from three core groups to two but have added follow-up outpatient group psychotherapy opportunities.

Response to Pressures for Change

In response to these pressures, the staff at the IPC went through a reexamination of their mission and goals and established a set of action plans to be used to guide the activities of the program over the next 2–3 years. To force process- and feelings-oriented group psychotherapists to work on this concrete task was a challenge, but over several hours of meetings we were able to develop a basic mission for the IPC program.

Several strategic planning meetings were held by the entire staff based on a model proposed by Caruthers and Lott (1981). The purpose of the strategic planning sessions was to attempt to project the nature and direction of IPC activities in the next 2–3 years. The strategic planning process allowed participation by all members of the IPC staff and demanded a focused, orderly, and analytical approach with an orientation toward the future. The initial steps were to identify major trends and issues that had influence on the program, both from outside the institution and internally. Through identification of these issues, the strengths, weaknesses, potential opportunities, and outside pressures were identified. It became apparent that analysis of both external and internal forces was challenging because of the rapidity of changes in the area of health care delivery. Nevertheless, a long list of the issues was produced and an evaluation of them allowed us to develop a mission statement, a set of goals, and action plans.

Insurance coverage of psychotherapy services emphasizes the use of preferred providers in the home community, along with stringent precertification restrictions. The availability of good psychiatric care in home communities has shifted our patient base to a more local distribution. In addition, departmental perceptions of future changes forced by a national movement toward "managed competition" have compelled us to reexamine our role in the overall service provided by the Department of Psychiatry.

We initially worked to redefine our identity, purpose, focus, and values, and we incorporated those ideas into a new "mission statement" for the program. The mission statement encompassed the maintenance of a multimodal diagnostic and therapeutic assessment program while providing treatment services to enhance interpersonal relationships, self-understanding, and adaptive skills. We expressed the desire to maintain a caring, supportive, and nurturing environment in a program that was of high quality and cost effective. We also indicated a mission to provide education to psychiatric residents and other health care professionals in group psychotherapy skills and to serve as liaisons to other areas of the department in group psychotherapy.

Based on this broad statement, we developed a set of goals to define directions and focus for our efforts over the next 2–3 years. They included providing treatment services to patients, providing services to employee assistance programs, teaching group therapy skills, creating more-focused groups, preserving the core intensive program, and enhancing the referral base through marketing of the program.

Finally, we established a long list of action plans with well-defined activities and objectives. The plans were circumscribed and sufficiently focused to allow specific targets and outcomes within a deadline. These included opening specific focus groups, expanding evening hours, establishing a didactic program, and monitoring cost effectiveness. This strategic planning exercise provided a working document that we hope will be broad enough to provide flexibility as well as a focus of action. Redefining our mission brought a much-needed cohesiveness to our staff and program.

Impact of Managed Care

The exercise of examining our mission and goals forced us to look at our future under managed care. Efficiency, quality, and outcome appear to be the watchwords. Certainly, the efficiency of the intensive group therapy format is beyond dispute. With increasing emphasis on efficient treatment, however, there is real concern that underlying issues causing symptom complexes may be glossed over in favor of a quick fix with medication or brief counseling.

It is our impression that providing 70–100 hours of active therapy over a period of 2–3 weeks allows a rapid breaking through of resistances and greater possibility for improvement. The complexity of interpersonal pathology requires a variety of experiences and sufficient time to permit its expression. The intensity and inherent efficiency of day treatment programs provide an opportunity for significant gains in a condensed time frame. Outcome studies (MacKenzie and Pilling 1972; Swenson and Martin 1976) indicate that improvement is sustained over at least a 6-month period. An important operational question that we have not been able to address because of the far-flung nature of our referral patterns is whether this positive clinical response translates into a reduced future need for medical care over longer periods of time.

The current national health care program proposals have major implications for a large referral center such as the Mayo Clinic. There is concern that an integrated service network, or managed care system, will restrict access to people who live geographically close and exclude those who are not members of the network. The institution is already anticipating an accentuation of integrated service networks by actively working to cooperate with other health care delivery organizations to establish regional networks. The presumption is that members of these health care networks will provide comprehensive services on a capitated basis. It remains to be seen whether this will place additional demand on our psychotherapy program, but it would seem to be a reasonable assumption that programs such as ours that can deliver psychiatric care to large numbers of patients in an efficient manner will be called on as models to meet an increasing demand for patient services.

With fewer medical students choosing psychiatry as a career (Yager and Borus 1987), there will not be a sufficient number of psychiatrists to meet the demand for psychotherapy services in the future. Expansion of the role and responsibility of the group psychotherapist to include assessment, individual and conjoint counseling, triage, case management, and consultation is necessary. The intensive group psychotherapy program model has the inherent efficiency and integration to provide excellent care with adequate supervision. All these programs must begin to systematically collect patient data to track outcome, and allow comparison with other treatment approaches.

A periodic redefinition of mission and goals appears to be helpful to maintain identity, productivity, and purpose in these rapidly changing times.

References

American Psychiatric Association: Diagnostic and Statistical Manual of Mental Disorders, 2nd Edition. Washington, DC, American Psychiatric Association, 1968

Caruthers JK, Lott GB: Mission Review: Foundation for Strategic Planning. Boulder, CO, National Center for Higher Education Management Systems, 1981

Hathaway SR, McKinley JC: Minnesota Multiphasic Personality Inventory. Minneapolis, MN, University of Minnesota, 1943

MacKenzie KR, Pilling LF: An intensive therapy day clinic for out-of-town patients with neurotic and psychosomatic problems. Int J Group Psychother 22:352–363, 1972

Orlinsky DE, Howard KI: Process and outcome in psychotherapy, in Handbook of Psychotherapy and Behavior Change, 3rd Edition. Edited by Garfield SL, Bergin AE. New York, Wiley, 1986, pp 311–381

Robinson LA, Berman JS, Neimeyer RA: Psychotherapy for the treatment of depression: a comprehensive review of controlled outcome research. Psychol Bull 108:30–49, 1990

Smith MH, Glass GV, Miller TI: The Benefits of Psychotherapy. Baltimore, MD, Johns Hopkins University Press, 1980

Swenson WM, Martin HR: A description and evaluation of an outpatient intensive psychotherapy center. Am J Psychiatry 133:1043–1046, 1976

Weiner MF: Group therapy reduces medical and psychiatric hospitalization. Int J Group Psychother 42:267–275, 1992

Yager J, Borus JF: Are we training too many psychiatrists? Am J Psychiatry 144:1042–1048, 1987

Chapter 6

Brief Day Treatment for Nonpsychotic Patients

Stephen J. Melson, M.D.

*O*utpatient psychiatric services have been offered since 1972 in the large multispecialty group practice setting on which I have based this chapter. The short-term intensive group psychotherapy (SIGP) unit opened in November 1975 in response to the need for a program of immediate intervention and support for those patients referred from within the medical center with moderate to severe somatic and psychological distress. Some 2,500 patients have been admitted to date. In this chapter I describe the program and provide an analysis of its cost effectiveness.

In 1986, the Virginia Mason Medical Center in Seattle started a health maintenance organization (HMO) health plan, which introduced more primary care activities and prepaid concepts into the traditional fee-for-service specialty referral practices. In 1990, the Section of Psychiatry and Psychology agreed to assume responsibility for the management and provision of mental health and chemical dependency services to the HMO population (Goldberg et al. 1992). The existing programs continued with a mixture of fee-for-service, HMO, and public welfare patients. The internal case management system devised for the HMO played an increasingly important role in the section's changing practices and serves as a model for enhancing practice efficiencies.

As the health plan grew to 42,000 enrollees by 1993, the demand for mental health services and benefits under the plan also expanded. Although limited compared with traditional indemnity insurance coverage, HMO service demands occupied an increasing proportion of the staff time of the Department of Psychiatry, finally reaching the current level of 40% of the psychiatrists', psychologists', and masters-degree-level psychotherapists' practices.

Program Description

In many a psychotherapist's view, there has long existed a need for an intermediate treatment format between traditional weekly outpatient group or individual psychotherapy and full-time hospitalization. This type of intermediate care would be group-based, making use of demonstrated efficiency of time and efficacy of treatment; time-limited, for the structure and pressure for change that this parameter provides; and applicable in a broad variety of clinical settings for a heterogeneous patient population. The SIGP unit was designed to meet these criteria.

More intensive and interactive than most day hospital programs, SIGP is designed to provide treatment for acutely disabled, chronically distressed, nonpsychotic patients. The setting in an outpatient medical office building avoids the expense, stigma, and restrictions of psychiatric hospitalizations. Discouraged, dysphoric, and somatically distressed patients are removed from the isolation of home and work environments that are unable to contain or nurture them. Support is coupled with intensive self-inquiry in daily psychodynamic groups and a range of auxiliary therapies that enhance and facilitate the group process. The program has six to eight patients in attendance at most times. Psychological goals of treatment are ambitious for an average 15-day (3-week) length of stay: beyond restoration of hope and a sense of self-competence from the enriched interchange and support of the group lies insightful mastery of psychological conflict or trauma that can allow new levels of functioning and prevent a return to old, self-defeating patterns.

The SIGP unit weekly program schedule is shown in Table 6–1. Core psychodynamic groups constitute the central focus of the program. They generate material that is refocused or reworked by auxiliary therapies and brought back to the core groups, where it receives further modification or validation. It is essential to have auxiliary therapies built into the program and in regular use, so that patients with differing needs and abilities can approach issues in a variety of ways: verbal, nonverbal, visual, tactile, or kinetic. A variety of these auxiliary therapies have been developed.

Table 6–1. Weekly schedule for SIGP Unit

Time	Monday	Tuesday	Wednesday	Thursday	Friday
8:30 A.M.		Patient's group	Videotape review	Videotape review	Anxiety management training
9:00 A.M.	Psychodynamic group	Psychodynamic group	Psychodynamic group	Art review group	Family group
10:30 A.M.	Break (staff session)	Break (staff session)	Break (staff session)	Break (staff session)	Break (staff session)
11:00 A.M.	Art therapy	Art therapy	Medication group	Psychodrama	Group prepares lunch with families and guests
12:30 P.M.	Lunch	Lunch (staff meeting)	Lunch	Lunch	
1:30 P.M.	Psychodynamic group	Film group	Psychodynamic group	Psychodynamic group	Psychodynamic group
2:30 P.M.	Break	Break	Break		End of week
2:45 P.M.	Discussion of program	Psychodynamic group	Anxiety management training		
3:00 P.M.	Videotape review				

Art Therapy

Art therapy (Thurman and Melson 1982) as practiced in our program involves introductory and advanced projects or assignments that explore internal conflicts and memories through drawing, painting, and the construction of objects. For example, patients construct elaborate personal masks. The masks are brought to the core group on Thursday morning for presentation and discussion. This nonverbal daily activity, pursued in its own quiet space and led by a staff therapist, becomes for many patients both a refuge and an introspective experience.

Focused Action Therapy

Focused action therapy involves reenacting the same issues and conflicts raised elsewhere in the program in a process that the entire group shares. This powerful psychodramatic tool is used each week by both patients and staff (two therapists are specially trained in the technique) so that in the course of an average 3-week (15-day) stay, most patients have the opportunity to serve in a variety of central and auxiliary roles.

For example, a 35-year-old professional woman was overwhelmed by intrusive images of her brother's death by drowning. She was able to use dramatic techniques to reenact the events of his death using other patients as participants. This process allowed her to move into working out her grief, which she had resisted for several years. Recent encounters with similar victims of drowning in the course of her work as an emergency room nurse had led to her psychological decompensation and inability to work. The key component for her recovery and return to work was found in this auxiliary therapy, which was reinforced by further efforts in psychodynamic groups and art therapy.

Video Profile Confrontation

Video profile confrontation (Alger 1971) is a video technique that uses natural facial asymmetry to explore conflicts in self-concept. Individuals are selected to work with a therapist and video cameras that project right and left facial profiles onto a split-screen monitor in front of the patient. This technique is particularly effective with dissociative and identity disorders.

Anxiety Management

Anxiety management is taught by a clinical psychologist staff member in twice-weekly group sessions. Cognitive-behavioral concepts are taught and reading assignments are given. Relaxation techniques and management of obsessive thought patterns and somatic preoccupations are practiced.

Film Group

The film group is held weekly. A staff therapist watches a selected film with the group and leads a discussion. This occurs early in the week, when uncovering/exploratory activities are encouraged. The films, both animated and acted, are evocative and portray common themes such as childhood trauma, alcoholic families, loss, suicide, seasons of life, and parenting.

Medication Group

The medication group is conducted by the attending psychiatrist or staff registered nurse at midweek. Patients learn about the psychotropic medications they are taking, discuss treatment and side effects, and have their dosages adjusted.

Family Group

A family group is held at the end of each week for invited guests (e.g., family members or significant others) to participate in group work, add new material, and reconcile or reveal important new insights.

Videotaping

Videotaping of morning psychodynamic groups occurs daily. Later, regularly scheduled replays promote clarification and refocusing. These occur on several days of the week and are conducted by a staff member other than the group therapist. The goal is to use the self in the role of an observer.

The creative integration of these group therapy experiences produces a whole that becomes greater than the sum of the parts. Throughout, there is careful attention to individual and group treatment plans, with daily staff meetings and weekly full-staff reviews. Discharge and follow-up recommendations all contribute to the behavioral goals of symptom reduction, return to work, and reduced or more appropriate use of medical resources.

Program Management

Admission procedures and criteria include 1) a previous psychiatric assessment or diagnostic interview with a medical center psychiatrist, psychologist, or psychotherapist who refers the patient for potential admission; and 2) an interview and tour of the unit with the unit coordinator, often with a spouse or other family member. The coordinator initiates a file with demographic and insurance data, assesses the degree of urgency of the proposed admission, administers any preadmission testing, and assembles data (including assessment, working diagnosis, ratings, and tests) into a file that can be presented to an internal or external case manager.

Generally, the referring source determines the overall suitability of the patient for this level of care, noting the absence of psychotic symptoms, active chemical dependency, organic brain syndrome, or immediate suicidal intent. A Global Assessment of Functioning (GAF) Scale[1] score between 25 and 60 assigned by the referring therapist further supports the proposed admission. In this population, lower GAF Scale scores reflect serious impairments in communication, judgment, or daily functions rather than delusions or impairments in reality testing.

Reauthorizations for treatment are often required every 5 days by managed care operations. These are based on progress in attainment of treatment goals, which is reviewed and rated weekly in staff conferences, followed by communication of discharge and follow-up plans. Discharge plans are formulated in the last 5 days of attendance, in staff reviews, and in an individual session with a therapist. Attainment of treatment goals, return of functions, and the need to consolidate or maintain therapeutic gains are considered. The dropout rate is exceedingly low: less than 5% complete fewer than 10 days of treatment. The

---

[1] The GAF Scale is a revision of the Global Assessment Scale (Endicott et al. 1976) and the Children's Global Assessment Scale (Shaffer et al. 1983).

readmission rate is also in the same low range. Occasionally, a patient will require hospitalization while in the program, but will return to the program after a few days.

Patient Characteristics and Outcome

Demographically, individuals admitted to the intensive day program are predominantly Caucasian (94%), early middle-aged (mean = 39.3 years) women (78%), who are married (64%) or divorced (18%), and well educated (90% high school diploma or above). Forty percent have had previous psychiatric treatment, and 18% have previously attempted suicide.

Clinically, they present in crisis with a variety of intense anxiety, depressive, and somatic symptoms (Symptom Checklist [SCL]-90-R Global Severity Index mean t score = 75.2, with a range from 59 [moderate severity] to 81 [extremely severe, top of scale]). On the DSM-III-R (American Psychiatric Association 1987) Axis V GAF Scale, patients range from moderate to severe impairment of usual daily functions (mean = 48.7, with a range from 60 to 25).

Psychotherapy outcome studies in a clinical setting present complex practical and methodological challenges to the clinician/researcher. Patients often present with both a current precipitating stressor and an extensive history of trauma, loss, or abuse. The patients' current levels of distress and impairment, including suicidal intent and moderate to severe loss of daily functions, often preclude their being put on a waiting list or the use of less-intensive treatment options, which would enable them to be part of a randomly assigned control group. Lacking a comparable group program where treatment variables could be introduced or withheld, we have systematically collected standardized self-report measures and therapist ratings repeated at intervals, applied in a reasonably constant, structured treatment environment by a consistent staff.

A 2-year study of 60 consecutive admissions (Melson and Rynearson 1986) used a battery of standardized self-report measures. These consisted of the Minnesota Multiphasic Personality Inventory (MMPI; Hathaway and McKinley 1943), a global measure of pathology, and the Cornell Medical Index (Brodman et al. 1949). These measures were administered pre- and posttreatment, and at 6-month ($n = 60$) and 2-

year follow-up ($n = 50$). Therapists also conducted semistructured interviews at the 2-year follow-up interviews. These interviews inquired into the patient's current physical and psychological functioning, development and resolution of stressors, and ability to work. Ratings were made using DSM-III-R Axes IV and V, and the Global Pathology Index.

Given the design limitations previously noted, clinical findings using the patients as their own controls showed significant decreases in psychopathology, significant increases in positive social attitudes, and maintenance of most treatment effects over 6-month and 2-year intervals. For the 31 patients regularly employed during the year before therapy, mean working days lost due to illness declined dramatically in the year after treatment, from a pretherapy mean of 22.7 days to a posttherapy mean of 2.5 days. Forty percent of the 50 patients followed for 2 years had 5 or more hours of psychotherapy in the 2 years after discharge. These cases showed a marked bimodal distribution. About one-half used only half a dozen sessions over the 2 years. The other half, or 11 patients of the original 60, continued to be intensive users of psychotherapy services. This group consisted of patients with primarily Axis II diagnoses.

Therapist ratings and patient self-ratings tended to be very similar. An example of the repeated standardized measures of psychopathology is shown in Figure 6–1. This composite MMPI graph of 50 patients with depressive disorder (major depression, dysthymia) treated at the SIGP unit demonstrates statistically significant decreases in levels of pathology, and maintenance of these changes over a 2-year period. These encouraging findings suggest that the treatment philosophy of the program—to provide a substantial measure of psychodynamic, reconstructive psychotherapy attuned to each patient's central conflicts, as well as supportive care to restore previous levels of functioning, all in a short-term treatment episode—is as pertinent to a managed care environment as it is to fee-for-service systems.

Medical Cost Offset

The above-quoted study (Melson and Rynearson 1986) appeared to show a marked reduction in medical expenditures in the year after treatment. Unfortunately, difficulty in obtaining accurate accounting

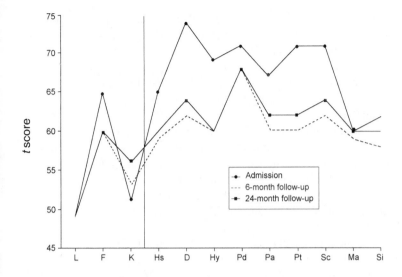

Figure 6–1. Mean patient scores on Minnesota Multiphasic Personality Inventory (MMPI; Hathaway and McKinley 1943) (*n* = 140). L = Lie Scale, F = Frequency Scale, K = Correction Scale, Hs = Hypochondriasis Scale, D = Depression Scale, Hy = Hysteria Scale, Pd = Psychopathic Deviance Scale, Pa = Paranoia Scale, Pt = Psychasthenia Scale, Sc = Schizophrenia Scale, Ma = Mania Scale, Si = Social Introversion Scale.

figures compromised the results. A second study was therefore undertaken when financial data of all medical expenditures over a 2-year period of all psychotherapy unit admissions from the medical center's HMO could be obtained.

A claims report detailing all medical expenditures for a 2-year period (mid-1990 to mid-1992) was obtained and analyzed for all 63 admissions to the intensive psychotherapy unit from the medical center's HMO. This cohort was chosen because complete and accurate figures were available that separated medical from mental health claims. These 63 patients admitted through HMO case management procedures represented 29% of total admissions (*n* = 218) over the 2-year period, which was consistent with the percentage of HMO patients in the psychiatry section's outpatient operations. Seventy-eight percent were women, slightly higher than the usual 2:1 female predominance in psychiatric practice, and the average age was 40 years, which was consistent with previous studies.

Medical expenditures for 1 year before and 1 year after the SIGP unit treatment episode were compared. Twenty-five patients (38%) had no medical claims during the year before or the year after their unit treatment.

Thirty-eight patients (62%) had claims for medical services the year before or after treatment or both. Age and sex differences between the two groups were nonsignificant (two-tailed t test). For these 38 patients, a considerable differential emerged. Twenty-seven of the 38 used more medical services in the year before treatment than in the year after. Total medical claims paid by the HMO for the year before treatment in the psychotherapy unit were $52,162. In the year after treatment, medical claims were $20,954 (Table 6–2). This was a statistically significant difference (two-tailed t test; $P = .015$). It should be noted that one-half of this amount was accounted for by a single patient who required cataract surgery.

Cost of Intensive Group Therapy

Cost to the HMO

The average payment per patient for the 63 patients in 1991–1992 was $2,615. This was for an average length of stay of 15 days, or 3 weeks.

Table 6–2.   Medical utilization in a prepaid health plan

1990–1992	n	Total claims paid	Mean claims paid	Standard deviation	Median	Range
1 year before SIGP	38	$52,162	$1,562	$2,904	$501	$22–12,410
1 year after SIGP	38	$20,954	$554	$1,866	$88	$11–11,414

SIGP = Short-Term Intensive Group Psychotherapy Unit.

Cost to the Patient

Most HMO contracts require 50% copayment for mental health benefits. Usually there are benefit limits of 10 hospital days or 20 partial hospital days, and 20 outpatient visits per year, with a cap of $1,000/year on copayments.

Cost to the Section of Psychiatry

The average cost of providing a treatment episode is $2,126/patient. This includes staff expenses for 1.0 full-time equivalent (FTE) Academy of Certified Social Workers (A.C.S.W.) therapist, 1.0 FTE program coordinator, 0.3 FTE psychiatrist, 0.1 FTE clinical psychologist, plus 22% benefits, plus one-twelfth of the total for staff absence coverage. Space and material cost per year, plus meals, supplies, and excise tax were then added to the costs of staffing. This total was divided by the average annual admission rate of 109.

Because these patients were selected, not randomized, for admission, and because no comparison group was available because of claims report limitations, results must be interpreted with caution. The higher mean expenditure for the 27 patients who used more medical services before treatment represented a few who had extensive workups and medical treatments. Patients tend to come to mental health services farther downstream in the river of medical services, if not actually having tumbled over the falls. Similarly, general medical service utilization during the follow-up year was highly skewed, with the majority of patients being quite low users.

The nearly 2.5:1 medical dollar expenditure for these patients in the year before entering the intensive day program compared with the year after is in line with other medical cost offset studies of psychotherapy (Budman et al. 1984, 1988; Holder and Blose 1987). Moreover, three large studies of medical cost savings of similar ambulatory mental health populations found that medical costs dropped continuously for up to 5 years after mental health treatment (Borus et al. 1985; Fiedler and Wight 1989; Holder and Blose 1987).

These results suggest that rather than seeking to curtail mental health benefits and discouraging their use by instituting high-percentage copayments, HMOs with capitated practitioner arrangements could save considerable amounts of physician and other practitioner time, laboratory expense, and hospital days. By identifying somatization, depressive, and anxiety disorders at an early point, extensive medical workups can be avoided. By providing intensive treatment for those with severe dysfunction, an immediate reduction in general medical utilization can be predicted. The studies quoted above suggest that this reduction is sustained over several years, well offsetting the actual cost of providing the treatment.

The Managed Care Environment

A new industry has sprung up in recent years around the need by major corporations and insurance payers to control costs in medical practices. Without debating the overall value of the current "managed care" companies and their practices, most therapists would agree that major improvements could be made in the way patients seeking help enter and work their way through the mental health care system.

Under the "old" fee-for-service model, initial contact, evaluation, course and duration of treatment, type of practitioner, and termination of treatment were often left to happenstance and the particular practices of therapists—not very different from the rest of medicine. There was little or no incentive to "sharpen" the process on the part of either patient or therapist. Some patients received prompt evaluations by appropriate practitioners, followed by specific courses of treatment; others saw therapists trained in an area different from that which would have specifically addressed their clinical needs; and still others never made the initial connection, their natural resistance enhanced by difficulties with a treatment system limited to two levels of intervention: inpatient care or weekly outpatient visits.

In the managed care model practiced by our mental health division of an HMO that now has 42,000 members, the emphasis is on open access, early intervention, and the efficient application of a series of treatment options so that the best use is made of the limited benefits structure. In this model, group therapies of various intensities and treatment orientations (educational, cognitive-behavioral, psychodynamic) are essential elements of care, along with brief intermittent treatment (Goldberg et al. 1992). A summary of the mental health component of our program is shown in Table 6–3.

Insurance and managed care company reviewers tend to focus on behavioral goals that are easily quantified and that discount psycholog-

Table 6–3. Utilization statistics for a managed mental health program (38,000 covered lives)

Utilization	1991	1992	1993
Assessments/1,000 enrollees	44.66	39.61	38.29
Inpatient admissions/1,000 enrollees[a]	1.74	2.06	1.67
Intensive day treatment admissions/ 1,000 enrollees	0.89	1.19	0.74
Average number of sessions for individuals receiving outpatient services[b]	6.50	6.30	NA

Note. The assistance of Paul Green in statistical analysis is acknowledged.
[a]Does not include 0.49 admissions/1,000 enrollees where benefits were exhausted before admission.
[b]Does not include medication evaluation and medication checks, whether performed by a psychiatrist or another medical doctor.

ical learning and awareness as unprovable. The old psychotherapy adage, "you can't count what really counts," certainly pertains to this dichotomy. Tensions between distant case managers and clinicians are rampant. In the internal case management structure we have devised, the two have an arm's length but collegial relationship. Clinically experienced on-site case managers are essential to this "new" (to fee-for-service practitioners) system. They provide triage, telephone evaluation, referral to appropriate practitioners or programs, and follow-up functions. The case managers ensure that the patient receives proper care for the level of impairment, complies with treatment, and eventually terminates treatment. This managing of care, rather than simply seeking to reduce costs, requires highly skilled individuals who can enhance practice efficiency and quality of care.

Quality assurance consists of reviewing the qualifications and professional activities of the clinical staff. Utilization review involves studying how services are used by patients and practitioners. These functions have become increasingly important standardizing activities in larger organizations. They are often best carried out by internal case managers. In designing an internal case management system within an existing group practice, it is assumed that management functions should be separate from assessment and treatment, and that practitioners should not case-manage their own patients. Masters-level clinicians

(M.S.W., M.A., R.N.) with sufficient experience to effectively triage, collect clinical and demographic information, authorize or deny coverage, monitor treatment plans, and process referrals will attain parity with providers of care and can develop working relationships with those providers that will enhance patient care.

Most of our case managers come from the ranks of clinicians. They developed a special interest in this work and trained on the job. In an internal managed care system where the case managers are on site, available to the practitioners, and included as part of a team that has the best interests of the patient as the primary goal, adversarial relationships are less likely to develop.

It would seem obvious that providing group psychotherapy for six to eight patients for 90 minutes, at about one-half the usual hourly individual therapy fee, would be a cost-effective treatment for all concerned. But if case managers are to be expected to turn to weekly groups or more intensive day programs in seeking the most efficient treatment, the half-century-old tradition of individual psychotherapy once a week for 50 minutes as the standard of care will have to be challenged. In our HMO in 1992, the average number of sessions for patients receiving outpatient individual psychotherapy was 6.3 sessions (Table 6–3). This correlates closely with the national average for HMOs (Group Health Association of America 1991). Consider the possibilities for staff efficiency and savings to patients and the HMO if even half of those sessions were group therapy offerings.

The benefit structure of many prepaid plans, our own included, does not yet provide adequate incentives to practitioners or patients. For example, a plan might offer a 12-session weekly group treatment plan that would count as 6 individual visits at half the cost of individual visits. This would support a trend toward seeing weekly outpatient groups as the first-order therapy for a higher percentage of the clinical population. Internal case managers would be able to offer such a service for patients with moderate symptoms before more serious deterioration occurs.

In our system in 1992, there were 39.61 new assessments, 2.06 inpatient admissions, and 1.19 intensive day treatment admissions per 1,000 enrollees (Table 6–3). The treatment day was counted as one-half of a hospital day for benefit purposes; however, its cost was less than one-third of the per diem cost of a hospital day. Thus, the true cost advantage was underestimated. The availability of SIGP can be a significant resource to the case manager. Patients can be transferred, through intensive case management, from inpatient to intensive outpatient status before using all of their 10 psychiatric hospital days—for example, following a suicide attempt. Patients experiencing a deteriorating course—for example, because of debilitating dysphoric mood, medical treatment noncompliance, pathological grief, or severe somatization symptoms—can circumvent hospitalization with intensive intervention.

The integration of a case management system into outpatient psychiatric practices, and the addition of SIGP as an intermediate level of care, addresses several treatment concerns: declining psychiatric hospital beds with sharply limited stays, limited staff resources along with limited psychotherapy benefits, inability to increase fees to compensate for increased costs, and the growing need for a level of care that offers both supportive and reconstructive therapy for progressively debilitated to acutely incapacitated nonpsychotic patients.

References

Alger I: Television Image Confrontation in Group Therapy, in Progress in Group and Family Therapy. Edited by Sager CJ, Kaplan HS. New York, Brunner/Mazel, 1971, pp 135–150

American Psychiatric Association: Diagnostic and Statistical Manual of Mental Disorders, 3rd Edition, Revised. Washington, DC, American Psychiatric Association, 1987

Borus JF, Olendzki MC, Kessler L, et al: The "offset effect" of mental health treatment on ambulatory medical care utilization and charges: month-by-month and grouped-month analyses of a five-year study. Arch Gen Psychiatry 42:573–580, 1985

Brodman K, Erdmann AJ, Lorge I, et al: The Cornell Medical Index. JAMA 140:530, 1949

Budman SH, Demby A, Feldstein M: A controlled study of the impact of mental health treatment on medical care utilization. Med Care 22:216–222, 1984

Budman SH, Demby A, Redondo JP, et al: Comparative outcome in time-limited individual and group psychotherapy. Int J Group Psychother 38:63–86, 1988

Endicott J, Spitzer RL, Fleiss J, et al: The Global Assessment Scale: a procedure for measuring overall severity of psychiatric disturbance. Arch Gen Psychiatry 33:766–771, 1976

Fiedler JL, Wight JB: The Medical Offset Effect and Public Health Policy: Mental Health Industry in Transition. New York, Praeger, 1989

Goldberg P, Melson SJ, Johnson M: Implementation of managed mental health care in a fee-for-service group practice. Group Pract J 41:47–52, 1992

Group Health Association of America: 1991 Sourcebook on HMO Utilization Data. Washington, DC, Group Health Association of America, Research and Analysis Department, 1991

Hathaway SR, McKinley JC: Minnesota Multiphasic Personality Inventory. Minneapolis, MN, University of Minnesota, 1943

Holder HD, Blose JO: Changes in health care costs and utilization associated with mental health treatment. Hosp Community Psychiatry 38:1070–1075, 1987

Melson SJ, Rynearson EK: Short-term intensive group psychotherapy for functional illness. Psychiatric Annals 16:667–692, 1986

Shaffer D, Gould MS, Brasic J, et al: Children's Global Assessment Scale. Arch Gen Psychiatry 40:1228–1231, 1983

Thurman W, Melson SJ: The making of masks in psychotherapy. Psychiatric Annals 12:1086–1089, 1982

Chapter 7

Group Therapy for Seriously Mentally Ill Patients in a Managed Care System

Walter N. Stone, M.D.

*D*ecreasing public funding and increasing costs of doing business have squeezed mental health clinics, which struggle to meet requests for low-fee or public-supported services. Funding agencies attempt to ensure that their monies are used as efficiently as possible and, as a consequence, have established priorities for services. One response has been for the public sector of the mental health system to turn to forms of managed care in an effort to contain costs and provide diverse services. Services have been prioritized, and among the populations targeted to receive an increased portion of public dollars are chronically mentally ill patients.

The interventions necessary to sustain chronically mentally ill patients in the community are considerable. Psychosocial rehabilitation is an integrative approach emphasizing the development of each person's fullest capacities through learning procedures and environmental supports (Bachrach 1992). The model acknowledges the need to manage the medical (psychiatric) elements of patients with chronic mental illness with fundamental respect for the individual, a considerable achievement from the period when patients were institutionalized for extended periods or for life (Munetz et al. 1993).

Bachrach (1992) outlined eight essentials of psychosocial rehabilitation: 1) individualization of the program, 2) focus on the environment, 3) exploration of an individual's strengths, 4) restoration of hope, 5) exploration of vocational potential, 6) expansion of social and recreational life, 7) active involvement of the patient in rehabilitation planning, and 8) continuing commitment. Appreciation of an individual's capacities and limitations because of illness, and awareness that social factors and psychological responses to illness contribute to an individual's impairment, helps define the place for group therapy. Group treatment can provide opportunities for patients to explore and share their reactions to their illness and to find ways of managing and overcoming the stigma associated with having a disabling mental illness.

History

The history of the use of therapeutic groups for the seriously mentally ill in outpatient settings grew following World War II, when patients conditionally discharged from long-term hospitals were treated in groups (Stone 1993). The patients in these groups were primarily diagnosed as having schizophrenia. The success of these groups before the advent of effective pharmacotherapy surprised clinicians, who were skeptical that patients could engage productively in such meetings. Initial therapeutic strategies based on psychoanalytic techniques were aimed at helping group members develop insight. These efforts were altered, and in their place more supportive/interactive techniques were used in which patients were encouraged to deal with problems of everyday living and to overcome barriers to satisfactory interpersonal relations.

Clinicians recognized that utilizing newer techniques only partially overcame some of the obstacles to forming a cohesive group. Expansion of group membership to include patients with other chronic illnesses, such as major affective disorders or disabling personality disorders, improved member interaction and enhanced group cohesion (de Bosset 1988; Lesser and Friedmann 1980).

The advent of effective psychotropic medications that partially controlled major symptoms moved treatment further away from an exclusively psychodynamic perspective. Groups were developed in which patients received their medication in a group setting. Although these groups provided opportunities for socialization and increased interaction, this component of the treatment was viewed as secondary to administration of medication.

A sparse research literature, which primarily focused on schizophrenic patients, generally supported the use of groups for the seriously mentally ill for the prevention of hospitalization and for the potential advantage of increasing an individual's socialization and quality of life (Kanas 1986; Keith and Mathews 1984). Comparisons with dyadic treatment favoring one or the other approach were inconclusive and were confounded by incomplete descriptions of the intensity, frequency, or type of either individual or group treatments.

Managed Care Considerations

Defining the boundaries of the seriously and continuing mentally ill population has proven problematic. Bachrach (1988) has proposed that chronicity includes domains of diagnosis, duration, and disability—the three D's. *Diagnoses* include a spectrum of psychotic disorders, affective illnesses, disabling anxiety disorders (e.g., generalized anxiety, obsessive-compulsive neurosis, or some phobias) in addition to severe personality disorders. *Duration* encompasses past and future considerations, and *disability* is measured against a standard of the individual's impairment in fulfilling appropriate social roles.

Containing costs for individuals who can need lifelong care creates quite a different problem than providing care for those who need less-extended services. Preventing costly hospitalizations or repeated use of expensive emergency facilities becomes a high priority. Capitation payment systems that allow for flexibility and individualization of treatment strategies are effective in cutting costs for the chronically mentally ill (Reed et al. 1992). Outpatient psychiatric care is considered palliative and supportive, and only in times of crisis is intensive treatment provided. Under these circumstances the development of a cost-effective and therapeutically viable group treatment program in mental health centers seems optimal. However, despite the potential that groups for chronically mentally ill individuals provide a cost-effective treatment, this therapeutic modality has not achieved widespread acceptance.

Systems Considerations in Developing a Group Program

Both clinical experiences and the research literature suggest that group treatment for the chronically mentally ill patient population is an effective therapeutic modality, but its use in public settings remains limited. Barriers to implementing group treatment for the chronically mentally ill are considerable. From a service delivery perspective, arranging for a group program requires a number of modifications of administrative procedures. Space requirements have to be altered to accommodate groups of up to 12 individuals; increased clerical support is necessary to process patients and to assist therapists, who have greater amounts of paperwork per unit of treatment contact. Because most clinicians are not well trained in group modalities, additional expense is incurred in order to provide training and supervision. Administrative creativity is required to support group therapists as they embark on a new enterprise, often with considerable trepidation.

Clinicians often are reluctant to conduct groups composed of chronically mentally ill patients. Therapists, under pressure to maintain productivity goals, are aware of the increase of time-consuming administrative demands in caring for 8–12 patients. They hesitate to assume the responsibility for groups without appropriate productive rewards. In addition, many "good" candidates for group psychotherapy are also "easy" patients to care for individually. Therapists are reluctant to refer those patients to group treatment and be assigned new, more difficult cases as replacements.

Therapists trained in the individual psychotherapy tradition do not consider the possibility of group therapy at the patient's initial entry point, and patients rarely request it. If clinicians consider referral for group therapy, they generally have not had training in how to help patients to accept that referral. There are additional systems elements that go beyond the clinician's lack of experience in working with the seriously mentally ill in groups. Therapists need to see themselves as effective professionals. Embarking on a new enterprise can undermine their sense of clinical competence, which further contributes to their reluctance to assume the challenge of group leadership (Stone 1991).

Case managers, who generally have the most contact with their patients, have less background than most clinicians in considering referral to groups. A degree of persistence and tact on the part of the case manager is necessary in the face of an individual's reluctance to attend group meetings. Those patients who lead an isolated, lonely, and quiet existence and who can benefit from the interaction provided in groups are overlooked as potential candidates. In some settings, regulations explicitly restrict case managers from referring patients for individual or group psychotherapy to 25% or less of their caseload. This limitation is another attempt at cost savings that serves as a barrier to patients entering group treatment.

Patients also resist entering a group. They may not be able to articulate the goals that can be achieved by belonging to a group and may enter to please a referring clinician (McIntosh et al. 1991). It is very unusual for seriously mentally ill patients to request group treatment, despite their generally positive experience of belonging to and participating in groups in hospital settings. Ill-prepared therapists are not equipped to help patients enter a group in the face of a patient's ambivalence.

These are only a few of the elements in a system involving the treatment context, the clinician, and the patient that require attention in order to improve the likelihood of developing a successful group program.

The Cincinnati Group Program for the Chronically Mentally Ill

Central Psychiatric Clinic is the publicly supported outpatient clinic for the Department of Psychiatry of the University of Cincinnati in Cincinnati, Ohio. It is organized into four major divisions: adults, children, forensic, and supportive treatment service (STS). This latter division is for patients certified by the State of Ohio as seriously mentally ill. The STS serves about 500 patients; approximately 100 individuals in this division are enrolled in the group program. The patient population is diverse, with only a segment of those enrolled diagnosed as having schizophrenia. Many patients have affective illnesses or debilitating personality disorders, often in combination with other illnesses. Patients with primary substance abuse are not accepted into the STS.

The division, headed by a nurse clinician/administrator, has a multidisciplinary clinical staff composed of part-time psychiatrists, psychologists, nurses, and social workers. Psychiatric residents and social work trainees contribute a significant portion of the treatment services. Case management is available for most individuals, and clinical staff are divided into teams to provide for treatment continuity.

The emphasis of the group program is continuing therapy groups composed of a spectrum of chronically mentally ill individuals. Time-limited psychoeducational groups and symptom focus groups are conducted when clinical needs arise.

Treatment Goals and Group Structure

In concert with a rehabilitation focus in the context of managed care, a primary goal of group treatment is the provision of a supportive environment in which members' illnesses become stabilized, thereby reducing the need for emergency or hospital services. An additional aim is to assist patients to fulfill their own potential and to more effectively manage their lives. Through interpersonal relationships established in the group, individuals feel supported and learn new coping strategies. The strategy of continued support is used as a vehicle for patients to generalize their group learning into the outside setting and improve their quality of life. For a small proportion of the patients, a return to the paid work force, usually in part-time positions, is a realizable goal. Others are able to manage volunteer positions, which they find gratifying. A large segment of the STS patients, however, remain unemployed, with little expectation of returning to the work force. They have little structure or routine to their lives outside the tasks of daily living. They may require services throughout their lifetime in order to maintain their functional level. Change, if it takes place, occurs over many years.

Our STS groups are structured to fit the needs of this population. Attendance in groups of chronically mentally ill patients is erratic, despite reminders such as pregroup meeting letters or phone calls. Similar contacts are made after missed appointments (McGee 1983). In general, groups composed of seriously ill patients develop a core of regulars and a peripheral subgroup of intermittent attendees (de Bosset 1982). The intermittent attendees can be emotionally involved in the treatment process, but for a variety of dynamic and reality reasons, they choose not to attend regularly.

Our STS groups are composed of patients with psychotic illness as well as those with chronic dysfunction who are not psychotic. A significant advantage of conducting heterogeneous groups is the tendency for the nonpsychotic patients to be more empathic and to have somewhat greater social awareness than the schizophrenic individuals. Psychotic patients can perceive unrecognized dynamic meanings in others' statements or behaviors, but often cannot effectively communicate their understanding. The mixture of members with a variety of diagnoses enhances the interaction and capitalizes on the strengths each person brings to the group.

The flexibly bound model (McIntosh et al. 1991) was developed in response to this nontraditional group composition. The basic element in the model is empowering patients with the option of choosing how frequently they will attend. On agreeing to enter a group, patients are initially requested to attend four consecutive sessions. Following this initial period, the therapist and patient together decide, in the group, the frequency with which the patient wishes to attend within constraints of from once a week to once a month. This arrangement creates a base for further collaboration between patient and therapist. It enables patients to be more active and responsible participants in their treatment. The therapists also benefit from this format, because they neither feel "pressured" to have each member attend every session, nor feel less successful as clinicians with a group that does not develop a traditional cohesiveness in which all patients are expected to attend each session. A drawback of this approach has been a tendency to accept intermittent attendance and to not ask the patient to do more.

Other structural elements that contribute to the success of our STS group program is the staffing pattern. Almost all groups are co-led by a permanent staff member, usually a nurse or a psychologist, and a trainee, usually a psychiatric resident, who will remain with the group for 1 or possibly 2 years. Permanent staff provide long-term continuity for the group and have an important teaching function for the neophyte therapist. The staff member's recognition of the new clinician's progress during the apprenticeship serves to counterbalance the frustration he or she experiences with the minimal change that takes place in the patient population. Observing the neophyte's development helps the senior clinician maintain interest and prevent burnout.

With few exceptions, our STS groups are structured to meet weekly for 45 minutes, followed by 15 minutes to review medication. The presence of a physician cotherapist facilitates this process. When a psychiatrist is not part of the treatment team, arrangements are made for a physician to meet with the group during this final segment to manage medication needs. During this period, in compliance with managed care regulations, treatment goals are reviewed with each patient and updated goals are signed by both the patient and the therapist. The review potentially provides an opportunity for a more-detailed exploration of the patient's specific activities than are reflected in the treatment goals. For instance, a goal for a patient is to attend structured activities outside the home on a weekly basis. This might be discussed during the group sessions, but detailed examination of the nature and regularity of such activities is undertaken during the review. If the review is conducted conscientiously rather than in a perfunctory manner (an all-too-common occurrence), both patient and therapist are afforded an opportunity to assess the patient's change.

Therapeutic change is variable. At times patients regress, with emergence of disturbed behavior or psychotic thinking. During these periods, private appointments are available. Optimally, individual sessions are limited to periods of crisis, and treatment is continued in the group. Each patient receives individualized attention during a periodic review process, which can function as a substitute for individual sessions.

Group Dynamics and the Treatment Process

Groups for the chronically mentally ill develop along the same general pattern described for groups of higher-functioning individuals, although not all stages are traversed. Initially, members may be preoccupied with their inner worlds and have only minimal emotional contact with others. Gradually, patients become more focused on "receiving" from the therapist, and many dependency issues are addressed during this phase. Concomitantly, members react to one another's comments by reciting similar experiences. They do not directly interact, but respond to others' comments as a stimulus to tell their own story. This process is similar to children's parallel play. The subsequent group development is one of member-to-member collaboration. Patients seem more in tune with one another's affective states; they explore problem-solving strategies, which can include direct advice. Interaction is not so dependent on the clinician's stimulation (Stone 1993).

The therapist's tasks are linked to the group's developmental stages. In the initial phase, the therapist needs to be actively reaching out to quiet individuals, containing dominating patients, or—if communication is garbled—clarifying what is being said. A passive stance on the part of the therapist promotes regression, and patients remain in their own self-protective cocoons. Therapist activity encourages patients to link to the therapist. Within the context of the patient's dependency, the therapist can make linkages between the patients' associations—that is, they share similar needs for care, trust, support, or reliability. The strategy is to prevent each person from feeling isolated and alone—a singleton status (Agazarian 1989).

In the process of identifying themes that link dyads, the therapist can cautiously generalize the themes to include the entire group, thereby promoting parallel associations. Movement into the succeeding developmental stage is facilitated by the therapist's identification of themes and active "appreciation" (positive reinforcement) of members' nascent emotional attunement with one another. In this manner, the clinician makes use of the members' needs to please the authority to empathically support a useful behavior.

One of the major therapeutic tasks is management of a patient's affect. There are recurrent themes that preoccupy members of chronic groups. These include fears of and wishes for intimacy, fears of decompensation and recurrence of their major symptom states, concerns about physical safety and health (a considerable portion of chronically mentally ill patients have their medical needs underserved), and anxiety about expressions of hostility. This anxiety is particularly evident in the manner in which patients avoid or suppress hostile feelings within the group, although angry affects can be directed at abuse from the "system" or from the family. Loneliness and sadness are easier feelings to address, and the therapist can often make meaningful therapeutic contact by exploring the feelings of deprivation and loss that underlie angry feelings.

Sexuality is infrequently addressed in groups for the seriously ill, and often clinicians forget that sexual needs are part of their patients' lives. In most instances, the emergence of sexual themes in the group is a displaced expression of dependency needs. Too great a focus on those dynamics can cause the clinician to overlook the overt meaning of a patient's sexual drive.

The increased requirements associated with managed care also impact on the therapeutic process. Patients now may be required to complete a variety of checklists and to participate in setting treatment goals, which they must agree to in writing. In addition, patients are regularly required to document their financial condition in order to qualify for public assistance. At times this process is humiliating and confusing, because regulations are subject to change and are not evenly applied. In our groups, patients make frequent allusions or direct references to these administrative requirements that intrude into treatment. The current requirement in our system is that goal-attainment forms be completed every 90 days. In a group that has a census of 12–16 patients, almost every meeting is followed by discussion of goals with one or more patients. These requirements are experienced by patients and clinicians as an excessive intrusion of the system into their lives.

Recurrent administrative requirements become a lightning rod for expressions of helplessness in the face of bureaucratic regulations. The task of balancing administrative obligations against a patient's needs is not simple. Allusions to administrative errors at the welfare or Social Security office can be displacements of feelings about the treatment setting. Therapists often are bedeviled in finding a therapeutically beneficial intervention that addresses these feelings.

Experiences of dependency, helplessness, and anger present in patients' lives reemerge in the group transference. Patients are loath to address angry affects to the therapist. In oversimplified terms, they do not want to "bite the hand that feeds them." The decision to interpret covert meanings is based on the clinician's assessment of the therapeutic alliance and the group members' capacities to examine such processes within the group. Katz (1983) suggested that treatment progress can result from interpreting the conflicts in metaphor, which he believes allows patients to covertly feel understood and not overly threatened. There are occasions during which patients can work within the context of the treatment room. No guidelines exist, but in our experience, patients' responses to major boundary changes, therapist absences, addition of new members, or unannounced terminations can be addressed directly. In the continuing therapeutic dialogue, patients will inform the clinician of their readiness to examine their intragroup feelings.

Patterns of Utilization

No formal evaluation on outcome measures is available for our STS groups. Information regarding patients' rates of rehospitalization or use of other medical services suffers from the difficulty in tracking those who use a combination of private and public facilities.

Attendance and diagnostic information for all patients in five STS groups was obtained from clinic records. All five groups included a heterogeneous diagnostic population. Three groups (A, B, and C) had been formed in the past 5 years using the flexibly bound model. These groups were co-led by a staff nurse and a third- or fourth-year psychiatric resident; they met weekly for 45 minutes, followed immediately by a 15-minute period to review medications and to complete necessary clinic forms. The data were compared with similar information obtained for two groups that had been in existence for more than 12 years and that were not established using the flexibly bound structure. Group D had been singly led by a senior psychiatrist for more than a decade. Group E differed from the others because meetings were biweekly and were led by a single resident. Residents generally remained as leaders for this group for a 2-year period.

Attendance data for the groups were obtained over a period of several years. There was significant variability in attendance within each yearly period for all five groups. Optimal attendance is considered to be six or more patients, and only groups C and E succeeded in achieving that number in more than one-half of the sessions across sizable time periods. Group E, which met biweekly, was unusual in that it was the smallest group, with only seven members who were very regular attendees. Four of these patients were diagnosed as having schizophrenia and were receiving biweekly injectable medication, which coincided with the group sessions. No patient in the slightly larger group C received injectable medication. Average attendance of three or less patients suggests that the core group was insufficiently formed. This occurred in more than one-third of the sessions for groups A and D, and for nearly a quarter of the sessions for group B.

A primary feature of the flexibly bound model is the opportunity for patients to reach an agreement with the therapist regarding the frequency with which they will attend group sessions. Agreements ranged from weekly to monthly, and a number of individuals arranged to attend in an intermediate range, such as biweekly or two to three times per month. Twenty-nine patients were maintained on the rolls of groups A, B, and C during the final year of the study. Fourteen patients agreed to attend weekly, 11 in the intermediate range, and 4 monthly. There was a tendency for patients with affective disorders (bipolar disorder and major depression with psychotic features) and those with anxiety and personality disorders to agree to attend weekly or in the intermediate range (20 of 21 individuals), in contrast to a more uniform distribution for the patients diagnosed as having schizophrenia.

The attendance data were examined further in order to determine whether the patients kept their attendance agreements. The agreement was determined fulfilled if a patient had attended 75% of the agreed-on sessions. For example, a patient who had agreed to attend 50% of the meetings would be expected to attend only 24 of the 48 annual group sessions. Thus, to be counted as fulfilling his or her agreement, the patient would have had to attend 18 or more sessions per year. The expected number of sessions was calculated for each of the 29 patients. Twelve patients fulfilled their contracts as determined by the 75% rate.

Patients diagnosed as having anxiety or personality disorders were most likely to keep their agreements (7 of 10 patients). Four of 11 patients diagnosed in the affective disorders spectrum (excluding dysthymia) kept their agreements, whereas only 1 of 8 patients diagnosed as having schizophrenia kept the agreement, and that was for an individual who agreed to attend once a month. Patients in the affective disorder or schizophrenic diagnostic groups who agreed to attend weekly had very limited success in reaching their goals.

Change in frequency of attendance was explored, with the assumption that it reflected the patients' sense of engagement in the therapeutic process. Eighteen of the 30 patients who initially were enrolled in groups A, B, and C had continued treatment through the end of the study period. Seven were diagnosed as having schizophrenia, five were diagnosed as having affective disorder, and six were diagnosed as having anxiety or personality disorders. Patients were included in this tabulation who began treatment within 6 months of the group formation. Comparisons were made between the first and the final year of the study. A difference in attendance of 10% (representing slightly more than four sessions annually) was designated as a change. Only 3 of the 18 individuals increased their frequency of attendance across the two time periods, whereas 8 individuals attended less frequently. All eight patients who attended less frequently were diagnosed as having schizophrenia or affective disorder. Those individuals represented two-thirds (8 of 12) of the patients diagnosed in the psychotic diagnostic categories. Two of the three individuals who had an increased attendance were diagnosed as having personality or anxiety disorders.

Comparisons were made between continuers and terminators for the 56 patients who had entered groups A, B, and C. No differences were evident for patients diagnosed as having schizophrenia (8 continued and 9 terminated) and as having personality or anxiety disorder (10 continued and 11 terminated). Twice as many patients diagnosed as having affective disorder remained (12) as terminated (6). Most patients who stopped treatment did so precipitously, with minimal advance notice to the therapist or to the group. A small minority of individuals left after a moderate treatment experience (12 to 54 sessions) when they moved from the catchment area.

Discussion

Implementation of managed care in the public sector has lagged behind the private sector. The general questions posed by managed care with respect to time-limited therapy become altered when working with the chronically mentally ill population, who often require continuing treatment. Hogarty (1993), in describing the impact of family treatment and social skills training for schizophrenic patients, states: "Thus it appears . . . that when the treatment ends, its effects end" (p. 22). Depression, with its propensity for relapse, recurrence, and impact on family relationships and work productivity, can require extended rather than briefer periods of treatment (Klerman and Weissman 1992). No research data currently support superior treatment efficacy of dyadic psychotherapy over group psychotherapy.

Group therapy for the chronically mentally ill population has the potential to fulfill three major needs: 1) to meet the clinical needs of the patient; 2) to remain a satisfying professional experience for the clinician; and 3) to be cost effective. The clinical needs of chronically mentally ill patients include stability in their therapeutic relationships, opportunities to receive medication, and expansion of their social relations, which are generally limited. These patients learn that they are not alone with their illness and share their experiences in managing societal response to themselves as mentally ill individuals. Groups serve as a protected anlage of social situations. We assume that if patients engage in group treatment, they learn new ways of interacting in a satisfying manner. By achieving improved social relations, patients stabilize their illness and improve their functioning (Breier and Strauss 1984).

The structure of the flexibly bound group allows patients to choose their frequency of attendance—an action that serves as a partial remedy for the chronic powerlessness that they experience in treatment and in life. Regularly scheduled groups are respectful of a patient's time. The usual strategy in public clinics is to create a medication clinic and schedule a number of patients at the same time. The expectation is that a number of patients will be "no shows" and the clinician's time is used most effectively because there is a cadre of waiting patients. The result is that patients must wait for extended periods; the message is that the patient's time is not valuable.

Our study examines a patient's attendance as a measure of his or her capacity to engage in this form of treatment. Almost one-half of the STS group members were willing to attend their group on a weekly basis, and only a small proportion agreed to attend as infrequently as once a month. This suggests that patients had some intention of trying to engage in the treatment endeavor. Not unexpectedly, patients diagnosed as having schizophrenia appeared to opt for less-frequent attendance.

Our findings, however, were that less than half of the patients fulfilled their agreements. Overall, only 41% (12 of 29) kept their agreements as defined by attending 75% of the scheduled sessions. Just over one-quarter of the patients committing to weekly attendance fulfilled that agreement; all of those individuals were diagnosed as having anxiety and personality disorders. If these pilot data are generalizable, the formation of a core group of regular attendees is severely restricted and is limited to nonpsychotic individuals. However, experience with group E suggests that schizophrenic patients *can* form a stable core group, particularly under circumstances in which they receive regularly scheduled injections of depot medications.

Although patients may not adhere to their agreements, there is evidence that they do become involved in group therapy. Eighteen of the original 30 members of groups A, B, and C remained in their groups for the duration of the study period. Among those who terminated were 6 patients who attended more than 20 sessions, suggesting that difficulty in initial engagement in the group was not the reason for their termination. For all patients entering group therapy, the overall termination rate of 46% was not substantially different from the early dropout rate in groups for higher-functioning individuals (Stone and Rutan 1984).

Patients diagnosed as having schizophrenia or affective disorder show a trend of less-frequent attendance over the years. This behavior may represent a lessened need for treatment on the patient's part, which is compatible with reports that, over extended periods, schizophrenic patients' illnesses stabilize (Harding et al. 1987). This finding has implications for the treatment enterprise because if some patients attend less frequently, additional patients can be added to the group rolls, which helps to maintain a satisfactory attendance at each session. Our findings show that among the three major diagnostic categories, there are no differences in patients' rates of terminating or remaining in treatment.

These results point the way for therapists to organize heterogeneous groups of chronically mentally ill patients. The flexibly bound model permits individuals to remain connected to treatment without sanctions because of irregular attendance. Moreover, the model also serves the therapist. Clinicians are in a position to discuss with patients their wishes in relation to attendance. Thus, if a person who initially agrees to attend weekly comes only biweekly, that circumstance is open for discussion in a nonjudgmental manner. If there are specific resistances to more frequent attendance, these can be explored. The therapist is in a position to renegotiate the frequency while the patient is present and does not have to experience the change as a failure.

An essential element for therapists to have a satisfying treatment experience is for group attendance to be maintained. Sessions with six to nine individuals present seem optimal, but this goal was achieved relatively infrequently in our STS groups, and sessions with three or less patients occurred with variable but considerable frequency. Several elements contribute to insufficiently attended groups. When the newer groups were formed, we initially anticipated that the rolls should range from 14 to 18 individuals. This estimate was based on the literature (de Bosset 1982; McGee 1983) and our own experience. A membership of this size, however, was not achieved for any of the groups. After initially establishing a membership roster of 9–11 patients, therapists were reluctant to add members. Early dropouts were not replaced, sometimes in the hope that terminating patients would return to the group. Group A experienced this problem when a substantial subgroup (5 of 9 original members) dropped out during the first 12 months. The therapists were reluctant to add new members because they hoped to recapture some of those who had left the group.

Another source of resistance to increasing attendance frequency occurs after groups develop a degree of cohesion and maturity. Therapists are reluctant to add new members because they anticipate that such individuals are "sicker" and would disrupt the group. This was evident in the resistance of therapists in group E, an unusually stable group, that lost several members over a period of 2 years. Although the roll decreased from 7 to 5, the therapist was slow to introduce new patients into the group.

Therapists express a valid concern that the increased amount of paperwork associated with managed care is a sufficient reason for limiting the overall group census to 10–12 individuals. The additional paperwork is experienced as a great burden. Reduction in the number of forms would be useful, but this is not the only reason for the limitation in the size of the groups. Attention to all of these elements can increase therapists' willingness to accept more members into their groups.

Our study supports the use of groups as a cost-effective treatment. The more than 50% retention rate for patients needs to be compared with that for the chronically mentally ill person who enters individual treatment. Moreover, there appears to be a trend for patients to use services less frequently over time, thus opening opportunities for additional patients to participate in group therapy. Despite the apparent advantages of group treatment, only 20% of patients in the STS program are enrolled in groups, indicating a continuing reluctance to fully use this therapeutic modality.

Further research is necessary to address changes in patients' clinical status. Our preliminary study addresses only attendance patterns and does not examine the more-detailed clinical course. We do not have information tracing the impact of a patient's hospitalization on group attendance. Some individuals terminated and others continued group treatment following hospitalization. We also are not informed about the impact of group treatment on the quality of life. Despite the emphasis of managed care on cost containment, we should strive to find treatments that optimize opportunities for a satisfying life experience for this population.

Summary

The place of group treatment for the chronically mentally ill in managed care is in its early stages. Groups have the potential for providing cost-effective treatment for these patients, who most likely will require treatment throughout their lives. The advantages of group treatment include more effective use of the clinician's time and increased therapeutic benefit for patients who have diminished social networks and limited social skills. Attendance patterns using the flexibly bound model suggest that groups composed of severely ill individuals with psychotic, affective, personality, or anxiety disorders can develop a stable core with satisfactory attendance. Therapists can anticipate that more than 50% of patients will remain in the group for periods extending over several years. Those who remain appear to attend less frequently, however, which can represent a stabilization of their clinical course with lessened treatment requirements.

As requirements for managed care for this population evolve, evaluation of group treatment requires more-precise descriptions of the patient population, the therapeutic interventions used, and the outcome, including measures of quality of life as well as cost containment. Attention must be paid to the time and energy demands made on group therapists as the tendency to require increased documentation and concomitant paperwork escalates. Finally, government and mental health organizations need to streamline administrative procedures to facilitate more effective group treatment.

References

Agazarian YM: Group-as-a-whole systems theory and practice. Group 13:131–154, 1989

Bachrach LL: Defining chronic mental illness: a concept paper. Hosp Community Psychiatry 39:383–388, 1988

Bachrach LL: Psychosocial rehabilitation and psychiatry in the care of long-term patients. Am J Psychiatry 149:1455–1463, 1992

Breier A, Strauss JS: The role of social relationships in the recovery from psychotic disorders. Am J Psychiatry 141:949–955, 1984

de Bosset FA: Core group: a psychotherapeutic model in an outpatient clinic. Can J Psychiatry 27:123–126, 1982

de Bosset FA: Comparison of homogeneous and heterogeneous group psychotherapy models for chronic psychiatric outpatients. Psychiatr J Univ Ott 13:212–214, 1988

Harding CM, Brooks GW, Ashikaga T, et al: The Vermont longitudinal study of persons with severe mental illness, II: long-term outcome of subjects who retrospectively met DSM-III criteria for schizophrenia. Am J Psychiatry 144:727–735, 1987

Hogarty GE: Prevention of relapse in chronic schizophrenic patients. J Clin Psychiatry 54:18–23, 1993

Kanas N: Group therapy with schizophrenics: a review of controlled studies. Int J Group Psychother 36:339–351, 1986

Katz GA: The non-interpretation of metaphors in psychiatric hospital groups. Int J Group Psychother 33:56–68, 1983

Keith SJ, Mathews SM: Schizophrenia: a review of psychosocial treatment strategies, in Psychotherapy Research: Where Are We and Where Should We Go? Edited by Williams JBW, Spitzer RL. New York, Guilford, 1984, pp 70–86

Klerman GL, Weissman MM: The course, morbidity, and costs of depression. Arch Gen Psychiatry 49:831–834, 1992

Lesser IM, Friedmann CTH: Beyond medications: group therapy for the chronic psychiatric patient. Int J Group Psychother 30:187–199, 1980

McGee TF: Long-term group psychotherapy with post-hospital patients, in Group and Family Therapy 1982. Edited by Wolberg L, Aronson ML. New York, Brunner/Mazel, 1983, pp 93–106

McIntosh D, Stone WN, Grace M: The flexible boundaried group: format, techniques and patients' perception. Int J Group Psychother 41:49–64, 1991

Munetz MR, Birnbaum A, Wyzik PF: An integrative ideology to guide community-based multi-disciplinary care of severely mentally ill patients. Hosp Community Psychiatry 44:551–555, 1993

Reed SK, Hennessy K, Brown SW, et al: Capitation from a provider's perspective. Hosp Community Psychiatry 43:1173–1175, 1992

Stone WN: Group psychotherapy with the chronically mentally ill, in Comprehensive Group Psychotherapy, 3rd Edition. Edited by Kaplan HI, Sadock BJ. Baltimore, MD, Williams & Wilkins, 1993, pp 418–429

Stone WN: Treatment of the chronic mentally ill: an opportunity for the group therapist. Int J Group Psychother 41:11–22, 1991

Stone WN, Rutan JS: Duration of treatment in group psychotherapy. Int J Group Psychother 34:93–109, 1984

Chapter 8

Outpatient Groups for Patients With Personality Disorders

Barry M. Segal, M.D., F.R.C.P.C., and
Rene Weideman, Ph.D.

*P*atients with personality disorders are prevalent in psychiatric outpatient populations. They are difficult to deal with and little has been empirically shown with respect to the value of various treatments. When Axis I disorders occur in these patients, better-established treatments are available—but for the Axis I instead of the Axis II conditions.

Personality pathology can be represented by a dimensional model rather than by the DSM-III-R (American Psychiatric Association 1987) categorical system (Livesley et al. 1989; Schroeder et al. 1992). Patients with personality disorders express various dimensions to severe degrees, such as anxiety, impulsivity, narcissism, social avoidance, and suspiciousness. They represent one pole on a theoretical continuum of the degree of expression of dimensions. Less-severe expressions, such as "neuroses," represent the midrange of the continuum. The least severe expression of the dimensions is healthy psychological functioning, which represents the opposite pole of the continuum from personality disorder. Because of the pervasiveness of the personality disorder in the total experience and behavior of these patients, their problems are resistant to change.

Long-term, intensive therapy approaches are attempts to produce deep and lasting change in the patient's life based on a fundamental restructuring of the patient's personality. Because these approaches are time consuming and very uncertain of success, long-term psychotherapy may be appropriate only for patients who are particularly suitable by reason of their level of insight or degree of personality cohesion.

In the managed care environment, briefer and less labor-intensive approaches are required. The goals of these approaches are different from those of the intensive therapies. Winnicott (1965) addressed this point by saying, "In analysis one asks: how *much* can one be allowed to do? And, by contrast, in my clinic the motto is: how *little* need be done?" (p. 166).

In our outpatient group therapy program, patients from all of the Axis II DSM-III-R clusters are treated in a variety of groups, but those from the dramatic cluster (borderline, narcissistic, and histrionic) are more prevalent among the patients referred to us. In this chapter we focus on patients with borderline personality disorder (BPD) and describe the specific group program we have developed for these patients.

Borderline Personality Disorder

Patients with BPD make up 13%–15% of psychiatric outpatient caseloads (Gunderson 1984). Despite problems such as significant overlap with other personality disorders, the validity of the diagnosis of BPD is supported by many studies (Gunderson and Zanarini 1987). The construct is currently being widely researched and is felt to be clinically helpful. These patients are described as having a high degree of expression of dimensions such as affective reactivity, stimulus seeking, insecure attachment, intimacy problems, and identity disturbance (Schroeder et al. 1992)

According to DSM-III-R criteria, the diagnosis of BPD requires the presence of five of the following eight features: unstable relationships, impulsive acts, self-destructive behaviors, emptiness and boredom, intolerance of being alone, anger, identity disturbance, and affective instability. In addition, psychotic features are frequently described in these patients (Gunderson and Kolb 1978).

BPD patients have a tendency of high utilization of health services resulting from their lack of control of impulses and their acting out through self-destructive behavior or aggression. In therapy, they form intense transferences to therapists and produce strong countertransference reactions. A variety of treatment approaches have been developed for these patients, including residential treatment, short-term hospitalization, long-term intensive psychotherapy, long-term supportive psychotherapy, cognitive-behavior therapy, psychopharmacological intervention, group therapy, and crisis intervention (Paris 1993).

Various theoretical descriptions of the nature of borderline psychopathology have been advanced. Many of the theories propose the concept of a split in the personality. Kernberg (1975, 1984) suggested that borderline psychopathology results from the failure of integration of good and bad self and object images. As a result of this failure, primitive defenses such as splitting, primitive idealization, and projective identification are prominent in the patient's functioning. Masterson (1981) proposed that these patients are fixated at the rapprochement stage of separation-individuation, between attachment and separation. Linehan (1987b) described three basic dialectics as central in these patients: vulnerability versus invalidation, active passivity versus the apparently competent person, and unrelenting crisis versus inhibited grieving. A common theme in these theoretical formulations is the notion of the presence of disparate aspects of an unresolved self.

Individual Therapy

Patients with BPD are known to be difficult to engage and manage in therapy. The course of involvement with these patients tends to be stormy and chaotic. Intense transferences and acting out through extreme behaviors such as suicide attempts and anger outbursts are well known in this treatment context.

Long-term individual psychodynamic psychotherapies of various types have traditionally been regarded as the treatment of choice (Nehls 1992; Waldinger 1987). A variety of models for long-term therapy have been developed relative to differing theories of psychopathology. For example, Kernberg (1968) recommended that these patients be treated with an approach that confronts and interprets the patient's negative transference early, whereas Buie and Adler (1982) believe that the therapist should provide a real holding environment for the patient.

There are few empirical studies of the psychotherapeutic treatment of patients with BPD and those that exist have methodological problems. Most are retrospective and do not include control groups. Only recently have explicit diagnostic standards been used. The results suggest that many patients drop out of therapy, and of those who continue, many do not make significant progress. For example, a retrospective survey of long-term psychodynamic psychotherapies with BPD patients in which the therapists were experts in the field (Waldinger and Gunderson 1984) showed that two-thirds of the patients did not complete therapy and of those who did, only 10% were felt to have had a successful outcome. Only about 50% of patients were likely to continue their involvement with therapy beyond 6 months' duration.

Group Therapy

Apart from theoretical positions on the issue of group therapy for BPD (see below), several authors stress the practical advantages of this form of treatment. Macaskill (1980) comments that in the British National Health Service there are large numbers of BPD patients who are offered treatment but there is a shortage of trained psychotherapists; the practical argument for group psychotherapy is thus compelling. Nehls (1991, 1992) points out that many BPD patients face financial limitations that make individual therapy too costly for them. The need for more-effective and economical treatment is thus obvious. She also cites authors who maintain that individual therapy is iatrogenic for some people with BPD. Klein et al. (1991) describe an outpatient clinic that is mandated to treat a target population of people with prolonged mental illness, the poor, and those at risk for psychiatric hospitalization. Serving approximately 450 patients, this clinic meets its mandate partly by conducting 15 outpatient groups, including an Axis II disorder group for severely disturbed, difficult-to-treat patients with personality disorders.

Group psychotherapy is recognized as being helpful in the management of patients with BPD (Gunderson 1984). Clinical studies report a variety of positive effects of group experiences, such as improved ego functioning (Kretsch et al. 1987), improved interpersonal functioning (Schreter 1981), and the development of a more benign view of self associated with a decrease in polarization in the patient's view of the therapist (Greene and Cole 1991). The group approach can be particularly appropriate in these patients because it can minimize some of the adverse events that typify their treatment in a dyadic relationship. The group dilutes the transference as aspects of the patient's object relations are divided among the members of the group and the therapist. As a result, the patient's regressive tendencies are lessened (Horwitz 1987).

Horwitz (1980) sees groups as useful in countering the narcissistic attitude of entitlement exhibited by many BPD patients: hearing about the experiences of other patients helps them to see others as whole individuals and not only as objects to be exploited or to provide gratification. The group situation, with its relative lack of privacy, discourages the development of erotized transference fantasies. Each patient is exposed to the explicit or implicit variety of other group members' views of the therapist. This range of perspectives somewhat prevents unstable alternations between devaluation and overvaluation of the therapist.

An aspect of group therapy that seems specifically suited for BPD patients is the observation that they are able to accept feedback, such as advice, empathy, or confrontation, more readily from other patients than from the therapist (Clarkin et al. 1991). It appears that they are particularly sensitive to relationships in which a power hierarchy exists. When the therapist speaks, a dynamic related to the therapist's position as an authority figure results in the BPD patient's vulnerability becoming more exposed. The opportunity to relate on an equal level with other patients includes the chance to take on roles that are not available in individual therapy, such as giving advice, empathically relating to the disclosures of another person, and protecting another person.

Investigators have attempted to establish the specific aspects of the group experience that are helpful to the BPD patient. The therapeutic factors proposed by Yalom (1985) provide a useful framework for assessing these aspects. In one study (Macaskill 1982), opportunities to be altruistic toward other patients and to develop insight were rated as particularly useful. In another (Nehls 1991), the patients found value in the sense of universality and in existential factors. These investigations of the factors that are specifically helpful enable therapists to develop more specific therapy approaches for groups.

Many forms of group experience have been used and most of these have been shown to be of some value. Group therapy may be best used as a component of a multidimensional treatment program (Lofton et al. 1983) that includes individual therapy either before, concurrent with, or after the group experience. Heterogeneous groups are favored because the presence of patients with more stable personality integration is stabilizing for the BPD patient. However, homogeneous groups have been used (Roth 1980) and can also have specific benefits. The forms of therapist orientation and styles of therapy in the groups have also been varied, including cognitive-behavioral groups, support groups, and task-oriented activity groups. Psychodynamic groups of various sorts are the most frequently described.

The particular therapeutic interventions made by the therapist in a group session are determined by the therapist's model. In psychodynamic groups, a key intervention is the interpretation of the patient's psychopathology and the group process. A particular focus on underlying narcissistic injury (Macaskill 1980) can have value; the therapist interprets the patient's anger as a defense against hurt. The role of noninterpretive therapist activity in these groups is also recognized as valuable because it allows the development and maintenance of the therapeutic alliance (Stone and Gustafson 1982). Nehls (1992) showed that in successful group treatment of BPD patients, the most frequently used interventions were giving and seeking information.

The nature of BPD pathology, with its inherent instability and oscillations between disparate representations, creates specific problems for group therapy and the strategy used must address these. Klein et al. (1991) suggested that the use of group therapy in the treatment of BPD patients requires attention to aspects such as acting out, splitting dynamics, countertransference issues, setting limits, maintaining a functional clinical team, and erotization of relationships. They suggest that the group program include the involvement of other treaters besides the therapists, availability of supervision, attention to group composition, and an approach that addresses the integration of disparate representations of self and other.

Empirical Studies

There are few empirical studies of the value of group therapy for BPD patients. Dialectical behavior therapy (Linehan 1987a, 1987b, 1987c), including group therapy, has been shown in a randomized, standardized trial to be helpful. This new and distinctive approach combines the explicit problem-solving and overt skill-training focus of behavior therapy with a viewpoint and set of practices derived from dialectical reasoning in philosophy: "change and, therefore, growth occur as a result of opposition between contradictory, but interacting forces (thesis and antithesis) and their continual reconciliation on a higher level (synthesis). . . . the task of the therapist is to facilitate change by highlighting both aspects of the dialectical oppositions, and fostering their successive reconciliations and resolution at increasingly more functional levels" (Linehan 1987c, p. 153). Linehan names and describes three dialectical oppositions, or poles: 1) emotional vulnerability versus invalidation, 2) active passivity versus the apparently competent person, and 3) unrelenting crises versus inhibited grieving. Specific skills in areas such as emotion regulation, interpersonal effectiveness, and distress tolerance are taught in structured psychoeducational groups. In concomitant individual therapy, the patient is helped to integrate these skills into daily life. Patients attend skill-training groups for at least 1 year and then are offered a continuing supportive-expressive group to reinforce the application of the skills.

A second randomized trial compared individual psychotherapy with a specific form of group therapy (Clarkin et al. 1991) based on an approach termed "relationship management" (Dawson 1988; Dawson and MacMillan 1993). Early findings from this trial show that the group experience was as effective as the individual therapy, but that the patients in group therapy were more compliant with the treatment.

Concept of Relationship Management

This approach uses a concept of BPD pathology that emphasizes the presence of an unstable split between conflicting poles of the self system. This split separates two fundamental states of the self—competent and incompetent. We use the term *incompetence* to refer to expressions of vulnerability, weakness, and victimization. We use the term *competence* to refer to expressions of mastery over issues and giving advice. These states are manifested in an oscillating pattern of self-expression in which there is a discontinuity between opposing states of feeling and behaving—as one who can cope with life versus one who is unable to cope. The oscillations occur in reaction to the interpersonal context that the patient is experiencing at any particular moment. The unstable self system is overly "context bound" (Dawson 1988). The context is based on the role positions taken by others who interact with the patient.

The relationship management approach emphasizes the idea that the BPD patient is particularly vulnerable to feeling that the therapist has taken a dominant or controlling role, which predisposes the patient to experience himself or herself as incompetent. This dynamic can occur when the therapist is not neutral; for example, when the therapist takes the role of knowing more than the patient by interpreting the patient's behavior.

The aim of the approach is to minimize the tendency for the therapist to intensify the pattern of oscillation of self states that occurs when the therapist adopts an authority role—that is, a role experienced by the patient as dominant and controlling. The therapist in this model attempts to remain neutral and nondirective. Appropriate interventions include expressions of uncertainty, reflection, and interest and empathy. In the group setting, the therapist does facilitate interaction. By attempting to avoid making interpretations of the patient's psychopathology or the group process, the therapist avoids the misuse of both support and confrontation that are typical therapist responses to the tasks of therapy with this population (Adler and Buie 1972).

The aim of our approach is to provide cost-effective management that stabilizes the patients' chaotic patterns. This is consistent with literature that suggests that the gains these patients make in psychotherapy tend to be behavioral rather than characterological (Gunderson 1984). Thus, in this type of treatment of patients with BPD, the goal is not cure or major characterological change; rather, the interventions are aimed at management and reducing clinical service use.

Applying Relationship Management in Groups

We offer an open, long-term relationship management group to patients diagnosed as having BPD. The diagnosis is made at the time of initial assessment in our program when the patient is interviewed by a team clinician and by a psychiatrist. Diagnoses are made on the basis of the DSM-III-R criteria for BPD. Patients who accept the idea of coming to the group attend an initial monthly pregroup session where new patients meet each other and the therapists, and are informed of the system operating in the group.

The patients are told that they may attend as often or as infrequently as they choose, and that when they first come they will be joining a group of people who have been members for varying lengths of time. We inform them that we do not object to them having other therapy while they are members of the group. The group is described as a place where people work together to try to help themselves. The limits described to the patients are that the group is a place to talk about feelings but not to act them out. They are told that because the group needs to be a place where people can feel safe, aggressive interactions such as physical threats, loud yelling, or extreme hostile attacks are not permitted. Following the pregroup meeting, the patients join the ongoing group at its next meeting.

Between 8 and 12 patients are referred to the group each month. Approximately six to eight of them usually attend the pregroup session. Of these, four to six may attend the group at the following session or at some later session. The session at which the new patients enter the group is usually attended by about 12 patients.

The attendance at each session is variable. The group has a core made up of patients who are attending regularly or who have attended over an extended period. The core tends to fluctuate somewhat from week to week, and to undergo major changes on approximately a 6-month cycle.

The group has a high dropout rate. Some patients never return after the first session and some stop coming after three to five sessions. The patients who drop out include those who tend to drop out of all treatments. The system we use does not resist this process. Patients leave with the understanding that they can return at any time. It has been our clinical impression that for a number of these patients, the knowledge that the group is available has in itself had a stabilizing effect. It is as if the possibility of returning serves a containing function.

About 30% of those patients who attend at least one session after the pregroup session become regular attendees and many of them stay in the group for up to 6 months. About 15% become intermittent attendees and continue coming for a period of months. Of the long-term members, a small proportion continue attending beyond 1–2 years. Some members who participated as core group members for months before discontinuing their attendance have returned to join the core group again. The core group at the time of their return may be composed of a different group of patients compared with the earlier phase of the patient's involvement.

At any particular group, the membership tends to be made up of about 50% regulars, 30% intermittent attendees, and 20% new members. The average attendance at the group sessions is now 8–12 patients. In the sessions, the therapists attempt to restrict their interventions to those congruent with the relationship management model. Some of the clinical issues can be illustrated with a vignette.

A 45-year-old woman first attended the group wearing a pair of dark sunglasses. She did not speak and did not return to the group for

3 months. When she returned, she was again wearing dark sunglasses and did not speak. She went on to attend intermittently for a period of approximately 4 months, during which the issue of her sunglasses was raised by other members. She revealed that at the age of 26 she had decided to always wear sunglasses except at home and claimed to have done so ever since. Feedback that the sunglasses made it hard for other patients to see how she was feeling led to disclosures of her shame and self-doubt and the sense of protection she felt behind the sunglasses.

She began to attend the group regularly when she made a decision to use the group to overcome her need to wear sunglasses. Each week she wore a lighter pair than the week before (she had a large collection) until the session in which she took off her sunglasses and cried bitterly, saying little. Following this session, she did not come to the group for many weeks; she returned to an intermittent attendance pattern, which she continued for 2 years. Over that time, she gradually revealed her history and her current way of living, and at times would tell the other group members of the benefits of the group in her life.

de Bosset (1982) described the core group as a "stable and constant nucleus" that functions as the "stabilizer and catalyst of the larger group." He described three diagnostically heterogeneous open long-term groups for patients with schizophrenia, affective disorders, and a variety of other diagnoses. In each group, the core group contained four to six patients who attended for years. The core group was also an open group in that some members terminated when they had made progress; their place in the core group was taken by a new member or a peripheral member.

The core group of patients in our BPD group has much in common with those described by de Bosset (1982), but some specific features, such as the variability in membership from week to week and the fairly rapid rate of turnover of the membership, are related to the nature of BPD pathology. The average duration of membership in the core group we are describing is less than 1 year.

We observe that many patients tend to reveal themselves directly through disclosures that other kinds of patients find premature. In this group, however, dramatic personal revelations within minutes of first acquaintanceship are regarded not only without surprise, but with a feeling of recognition. The group discussions tend to focus on typical themes, such as impulsivity and its consequences, the tendency to experience strong anger, variability of affect, relationship breakdown, lack of direction, self-destructive behavior, feelings of emptiness, and histories of abuse and adversity.

The organizing perspective we take is that the patients relate through a specific interactional pattern that involves the patient's adopting one of the two major stances—competence versus incompetence. The particular stance adopted varies with the interpersonal context within the group. A patient may adopt opposing stances over a period of weeks, from week to week, or within a session.

The interaction around one of the themes is made up of a two-sided dialogue in which some patients adopt incompetent positions and some adopt competent positions. Examples of an incompetent type of expression would be "Last night I started breaking plates in the kitchen, I was so mad" or "I feel like I always get neglected like I was in my childhood." Examples of competent expressions would be "Last night I was mad enough to break plates, but I didn't, so I think being in the group has helped me" and "I've been trying to forgive my parents and I think it helped me to stop thinking about them so much."

In response to a statement of incompetence (e.g., "Today I've been feeling like taking an overdose") another patient will respond with either an incompetent statement (e.g., "I know how you feel because every time I drive across a bridge I think about driving over the edge") or with a competent response (e.g., "Thinking about suicide doesn't get you anywhere. You should find something else to focus on.").

In each session, there is an unstable balance between expressions of competence and incompetence. In other words, the group process itself takes on characteristics of BPD psychopathology. The choice of the expression of competence or incompetence for any patient is heavily affected by the general pattern of the balance between expressions of competence and incompetence over the session. The balance is generally toward the expression of incompetence, but invariably some patients adopt the competent position in order to stabilize the session somewhat. The unstable balance works reliably to halt a pervasive slide into nihilism that is always possible.

Greene and Cole (1991) suggested that BPD patients prefer an unstructured setting in which they tend to "band together to create powerful larger-than-life enactments replete with themes of betrayal, blame and neediness" (p. 516). The intense interactions typical of our group sessions seem consistent with this. In theory, the interactions of BPD patients could readily lead to a breakdown in the group; for example, an angry encounter turning into a fight. In our groups, the therapists' model-congruent interventions counteract the tendency to intensify the interaction. The modulation that results from the interventions of the therapist enables the enactment to occur in a contained manner. For example, if the therapist responds to an excessive expression of anger from a patient without taking an authoritative stance, such as by empathizing with the anger rather than confronting it, the role of authority-enforcing-limits may be taken by another patient—someone the angry person can hear better than he or she can hear the therapist.

The therapist's nonintrusive accepting stance acts to stabilize and modulate the interaction, producing a containment that enables group members to tolerate the extremity of their experiences and disclosures. The intensity of affect is dampened rather than activated, as would be the case in an interpretive model. The amplitude and frequency of the oscillation between opposing self states is reduced. The group thus functions as a form of holding environment.

Expressions of incompetence allow patients to experience a degree of catharsis. When other group members respond by revealing their own related feelings of incompetence, patients have the experience of universality, of being in some way similar to other people and accepted by other people. Sharing feelings of incompetence allows patients to experience empathy for each other. Expressions of competence enable patients to experience being altruistic to others.

The therapist's role is to be consistent, interested, and empathic yet neutral. The challenges inherent in the management of these patients makes this a difficult stance to maintain because of the countertransferences evoked by the patients. Feelings of hopelessness, confusion, anger, and frustration can become strong at times in the face of the patients' intrusiveness. These pressures can lead therapists to make interventions that deviate from their own approach—so-called "off-model" interventions. Therapists' internal processing of their own responses may be an important component of the therapy because it helps them remain "on-model."

To help therapists deal with this aspect, we have observers behind a one-way mirror who meet with the therapists after each session to discuss the group. Part of their work is to see whether the therapists make interpretations or supportive comments or recommendations as opposed to interventions that reflect neutrality and nondirectiveness. When we identify interventions that seem "off-model," we attempt to understand the factors that may have led to these interventions and suggest alternative model-congruent interventions. The involvement of a number of team members, the postgroup sessions, and the rotation of therapists on an annual basis have served to maintain a functional clinical team.

An intrinsic aspect of relationship management is that it provides an alternative approach that reduces the tendency of patients to act out by decreasing the iatrogenic aspects of the therapeutic interaction. The approach to threats of acting out, especially threats of self-harm, is to disconfirm patients' expectations of engagement in an enactment. In essence, the therapist responds with the type of interventions recommended by the model, such as empathy (e.g., "You sound quite desperate"), facilitation of group interaction (e.g., "Does anyone have a response to this?"), or reflection (e.g., "You feel that you should do this"). Our experience is that this approach provides genuine protection against the danger of patients acting out in ways that are a threat to safety. The permeable external boundary of the group enables patients to leave without processing their departures and this may also limit acting out in the group. As McIntosh et al. (1991) pointed out in an article on flexible boundaried groups, when the expectation of regular weekly attendance for all patients is relaxed, both those who are present in a session and those who are absent from it are able to accept irregular attendees.

The relationship management model also functions to contain oscillating opposing states of self. Neutrality of the therapists appears to minimize splitting of the cotherapists into a good object and a bad object. Instead, there is a low rate of focus on attitudes toward the therapists or confrontations of or attacks on the therapists. The containment of the intensity of the interactions allows the group to shift its balance toward the competent pole.

The BPD group functions as a component of a larger clinical service. There are resources for providing psychopharmacological therapy by psychiatrists while the patients are in the group if necessary. Some patients are offered brief individual therapy prior to entering the group. Approximately 40% of the patients have concurrent individual therapy independently arranged and some have in fact been referred by individual therapists, who suggest that they attend the group concurrently with the individual therapy.

Although the neutral approach we have taken has served to maintain the group as an ongoing system with few adverse events, there have been a few times when the group has been faced with behavior that contravenes the limits. For example, one patient fiercely and persistently denigrated another and then stormed out the room, opening the door with such force that it crashed into the chair of one of the other patients. The offending patient was subsequently told that she could continue to attend only if these behaviors ceased; she angrily chose not to return. Patients who leave the session early are not pursued and the group continues in its usual fashion until the end of the hour. Latecoming is also tolerated.

We chose a cotherapy model because this affords some relief of the pressures of the interaction. We ensured that the therapists are always of opposite gender and found that erotization of transference has not been a major factor. The group is the center of a larger, fluctuating system of social interactions that take place among patients outside the weekly sessions. There is no prohibition on outside interaction. Erotization of the relationship between patients has not often emerged as a theme in the group.

At times, concern over potential for violence in certain patients has been expressed by therapists and observers. These concerns usually focus on male patients who have prominent narcissistic features. Although there have been incidents in which these types of patients angrily attacked the group process, the outcome usually was that they either left the group or changed their behavior to be more consistent with group norms. The example described previously of a woman who angrily swung the door open so that it hit the chair of another patient is the only violent incident that occurred in the 3 years this group has been functioning.

Patients who become members of the core group tend to come from the midrange of BPD functioning. This type of group experience seems less acceptable to BPD patients with high levels of functioning; such patients may be more responsive to interpersonally focused approaches. Patients with a severe degree of BPD features have been long-term group members, but usually in association with individual therapy. Although some of these patients have appeared to benefit, the ongoing intensity of their needs suggests that for patients at the extreme of BPD pathology, more comprehensive approaches are required. Patients with marked narcissistic features have also tended to become dissatisfied and have left.

Dealing individually with patients who do call or seek individual contact can be time consuming for therapists. Whenever possible, therapists respond to patients who call or seek individual contact by suggesting that issues be brought to the group, but there are times when individual meetings seem essential in order to assess the presence of an Axis I disorder or to deal with a complex issue. The neutral role of the therapist does appear effective in minimizing the amount of individual contact sought by patients.

Although it seems logical to assume that patients who drop out early benefit little from the group, our clinical impression of the dropout population is that there is a low rate of adverse reactions, such as hospital admissions and emergency presentations. The fact that they leave of their own choice, with the knowledge that they retain membership and can return whenever they choose, has a stabilizing effect in itself. It alters the usual pattern of breakdown of engagement.

Our clinical impression is that some patients make definite progress, reflected in the group by an increasing rate of expressions of competence. A small but consistent number of patients achieve a stable sense of competence and leave the group as graduates. Some patients seem to find the group stabilizing and attend at a particular frequency over a long period of time, using the group as a supportive, steadying influence. For others, the group helps to stabilize their functioning in a way that enables them to make a therapeutic engagement in an individual therapy elsewhere. Still other patients find little of value in the group despite fairly regular attendance.

The program described in this chapter is a cost-effective technique for providing management to a large number of patients. Our experience suggests that the group can operate without significant adverse consequences. A changing core group of patients uses the group for long periods and many others have a peripheral involvement, so that a total of approximately 30 patients are considered members of the group at any time. For all of these patients, there seems to be either some improvement or at least no harm done, which suggests that this type of approach has value in the managed care environment. However, if such a program minimizes the adverse aspects of treating BPD patients, it also minimizes the goals of treatment. A degree of stabilization in the patient's functioning is regarded as a good outcome. The therapist in this model must relinquish some of the roles most valued by therapists (e.g., offering psychodynamic understanding), and this can be difficult.

References

Adler G, Buie DH: The misuses of confrontation with borderline patients. Int J Psychoanal Psychother 1:109–119, 1972

American Psychiatric Association: Diagnostic and Statistical Manual of Mental Disorders, 3rd Edition, Revised. Washington, DC, American Psychiatric Association, 1987

Buie DH, Adler G: Definitive treatment of the borderline personality. Int J Psychoanal Psychother 9:51–87, 1982

Clarkin JF, Marziali E, Munroe-Blum H: Group and family treatments for borderline personality disorder. Hosp Community Psychiatry 42:1038–1043, 1991

Dawson DF: Treatment of the borderline patient, relationship management. Can J Psychiatry 33:370–374, 1988

Dawson DF, MacMillan HL: Relationship Management of the Borderline Patient. New York, Brunner/Mazel, 1993

de Bosset FA: Core group: a psychotherapeutic model in an outpatient clinic. Can J Psychiatry 27:123–126, 1982

Greene LR, Cole MB: Level and form of psychopathology and the structure of group therapy. Int J Group Psychother 41:499–521, 1991

Gunderson JG: Borderline Personality Disorder. Washington, DC, American Psychiatric Press, 1984

Gunderson JG, Kolb JE: Discriminating features of borderline patients. Am J Psychiatry 135:792–796, 1978

Gunderson JG, Zanarini MC: Current overview of the borderline diagnosis. J Clin Psychiatry 48:5–14, 1987

Horwitz L: Group psychotherapy for borderline and narcissistic patients. Bull Menninger Clin 44:281–299, 1980

Horwitz L: Indications for group psychotherapy with borderline and narcissistic patients. Bull Menninger Clin 51:248–260, 1987

Kernberg OF: The treatment of patients with borderline personality organization. Int J Psychoanal 49:600–619, 1968

Kernberg OF: Borderline Conditions and Pathological Narcissism. New York, Jason Aronson, 1975

Kernberg OF: Severe Personality Disorders: Psychotherapeutic Strategies. New Haven, CT, Yale University Press, 1984

Klein RH, Orleans JF, Soule CR: The Axis II group: treating severely characterologically disturbed patients. Int J Group Psychother 41:97–115, 1991

Kretsch R, Goren Y, Wasserman A: Change patterns of borderline patients in individual and group therapy. Int J Group Psychother 37:95–112, 1987

Linehan MM: Dialectical behavior therapy: a cognitive behavioral approach to parasuicide. Journal of Personality Disorders 1:328–333, 1987a

Linehan MM: Dialectical behavior therapy for borderline personality disorder: therapy and method. Bull Menninger Clin 51:261–276, 1987b

Linehan MM: Dialectical behavior therapy in groups: treating borderline personality disorders and suicidal behavior, in Women's Therapy Groups: Paradigms of Feminist Treatment. Edited by Brody CM. New York, Springer, 1987c, pp 145–162

Livesley WJ, Jackson DN, Schroeder ML: A study of the factorial structure of personality pathology. Journal of Personality Disorders 3:292–306, 1989

Lofton P, Daugherty C, Mayerson P: Combined group and individual treatment for the borderline patient. Group 7:21–26, 1983

Macaskill ND: The narcissistic core as a focus in the group therapy of the borderline patient. Br J Med Psychol 53:137–143, 1980

Macaskill ND: Therapeutic factors in group therapy with borderline patients. Int J Group Psychother 32:61–73, 1982

Masterson JF: The Narcissistic and Borderline Disorders. New York, Brunner/Mazel, 1981

McIntosh D, Stone WN, Grace M: The flexible boundaried group: format, techniques, and patients' perceptions. Int J Group Psychother 41:49–64, 1991

Nehls N: Borderline personality disorder and group therapy. Arch Psychiatr Nurs 5:137–146, 1991

Nehls N: Group therapy for people with borderline personality disorder: interventions associated with positive outcomes. Issues Ment Health Nurs 13:255–269, 1992

Paris J: The treatment of borderline personality disorder in light of the research on its long term outcome. Can J Psychiatry 38 (suppl 1):S28–S34, 1993

Roth BE: Understanding the development of a homogeneous, identity-impaired group through countertransference phenomena. Int J Group Psychother 30:405–426, 1980

Schreter RK: Treating the untreatables: a group experience with somaticizing borderline patients. Int J Psychiatry Med 10:205–215, 1981

Schroeder ML, Wormworth JA, Livesley WJ: Dimensions of personality disorder and their relationships to the big five dimensions of personality. Psychological Assessment 4:47–53, 1992

Stone WN, Gustafson JP: Technique in group psychotherapy of narcissistic and borderline patients. Int J Group Psychother 32:29–47, 1982

Waldinger RJ: Intensive psychodynamic therapy with borderline patients: an overview. Am J Psychiatry 144:267–274, 1987

Waldinger RJ, Gunderson JG: Completed psychotherapies with borderline patients. Am J Psychother 38:192–202, 1984

Winnicott DW: The aims of psychoanalytical treatment, in The Maturational Processes and the Facilitating Environment: Studies in the Theory of Emotional Development. Madison, CT, International Universities Press, 1965, pp 166–170

Yalom ID: The Theory and Practice of Group Psychotherapy, 3rd Edition. New York, Basic Books, 1985

Chapter 9

Managed Care and Managed Competition

Howard D. Kibel, M.D.

*T*he chapters in this book were written in the atmosphere of managed care. Mental health practitioners have become increasingly frustrated by reviewers who seek to limit payments for psychotherapy. In this cost-conscious environment, group psychotherapy seems to offer promise. Compared with individual psychotherapy, more patients can be treated in a group in a specified segment of time, so that the cost per patient is reduced. Group psychotherapy should therefore appeal to health care managers, particularly those who operate capitation programs.

Since these chapters were written, the scene has begun to shift. The United States is engaged in a debate over health care coverage. Change is on the horizon, but what those changes will be is uncertain. The future of health care financing cannot be predicted. It will be subject to political and economic forces that have yet to be revealed, and their effect on the financing of mental health care, including psychotherapy, is unknown.

There is general agreement that health care financing needs reform. Political pressure is building for a comprehensive overhaul of the system. The public has come to accept the idea that some sort of coverage must be available to every citizen. Insurance coverage no longer will be optional; it will be required. The plan for universal health coverage that emerges from this debate will revolutionize our thinking about health care. Although coverage may be limited at first, the system of the future will probably embody the principle that health care coverage is the right of every citizen and that it will be his or her responsibility to join some sort of delivery plan.

It appears at this juncture that mental health benefits will be modest. They will probably be subject to arbitrary limits, and practitioners may still struggle with managed care. Even within these constraints, the ground rules could change with the advent of so-called managed competition. The latter will force planners to consider mental health costs along with other medical costs and how the former affect the latter. In this chapter I review the previous chapters of this book in view of the changing methods of financing health care.

Background of Health Care Legislation

When Medicare was enacted into law in 1965, reformers of the day assumed that it was the first step toward universal public health insurance in the United States. However, powerful interest groups collaborated to limit its scope. An opportunity may have been missed (Marmor 1993). Since then, medical costs have skyrocketed. Between 1965 and 1985, the total for national expenditures rose 10-fold. In the 7-year period between 1985 and 1992, the total doubled. Estimates are that by the year 2000, even with current efforts toward financial restraint, total health care costs will again more than double (Health Care Financing Administration 1991).

There is widespread agreement in the United States that health care costs have risen to unmanageable levels and that far too many citizens have limited access to adequate care. The United States spends more on health care than any other country. The cost for health care for 1993 was estimated at more than $800 billion, or 14.9% of the gross national product, and it continues to rise. Although everyone acknowledges the need for cost containment, experts disagree about how this should be done. At the same time, an estimated 37 million citizens do not have health insurance and 1.5 million more are underinsured (Grinfeld 1993). Many individuals with adequate insurance are unable to advance their careers because changing jobs would mean a loss of insurance. Thus, there is a recognized need for insurance coverage to be "portable"—that is, to move with the individual from job to job.

Partially in response to these conditions, Einthoven proposed a system of universal health coverage that has come to be known as managed competition (Einthoven and Kronick 1989). The Jackson Hole Group, an informal group of economists, policymakers, and health care providers, developed the concept and put forth a comprehensive proposal. They viewed the problems in today's system as stemming from perverse market incentives that cause patients to seek more and more services, and that induce physicians and hospitals to provide ever more costly services. The group rejected a single-payer plan, such as Canada's national health plan, which would do away with private health insurance and make the government the sole provider of health care. This is noteworthy, because some experts contend that insurance companies and the current system of quality assurance and oversight consume as much as 24% of the total cost of health care.

The current trend among leaders in health care planning, particularly those in a position to influence national policy, is to contain costs by promoting plans for health care delivery that encourage competition among large groups of providers. Presumably, in order to attract customers (patients), these conglomerates would compete by using a variety of cost-containment strategies. This is the thinking behind managed competition. If allowed, health care providers could lower their insurance premiums or offer more services. Alternatively, they could enhance profits by economizing—that is, by reducing expenses. Large provider organizations are best positioned to do this. Planners foresee health care of the future being delivered solely by health maintenance organizations (HMOs) and other prepaid medical plans.

Managed competition would restructure the health care delivery system so that care is provided by organized health plans that compete with one another on the basis of cost and outcome. Health insurance purchasing cooperatives (HIPCs) would purchase comprehensive coverage for regional groups of small businesses and individuals. Large industrial employers would purchase their own. A national health board would be created to serve as a central governing body that would define a basic package of benefits and negotiate fees with providers, namely groups of physicians and hospitals. The actual negotiations could be regionalized. The package would be "portable," would cover every working American, would remain in effect during periods of unemployment, and could be extended to those who are currently under Medicare. Although it is said that Medicaid would be folded into this system, that would happen gradually and might be delayed by several years. The cost of including the indigent would be great, and for that reason, their inclusion could be vulnerable to political forces.

A few regional health alliances would be available to each consumer, who would choose one based on price, benefits, or personal preference. Large corporations would have the option to negotiate directly with insurers for their employees' coverage. Corporate alliances would exist alongside regional ones, but the economics of the two might not be the same. Those who govern regional health alliances would consider overall health costs, much like HMOs currently do. However, corporate alliances could be interested in the relationship of health care to work productivity and perhaps even to retirement costs. This, the economics of the two could prove to be significantly different.

Mental health costs have not been spared from escalation. In 1990 they accounted for 10% of total health costs, but already that percentage has increased. The rate of increase in recent years for mental health costs has exceeded the rate for health care expenditures in general. This is a consequence of several factors, the most important of which is an expansion of insurance coverage to psychiatric disorders. At present, 42 states mandate that health care policies include coverage for mental disorders and about 98% of all insurance policies include some mental health benefits (Mirin 1993).

A large part of the increase in mental health costs has come from increased utilization of inpatient services—specifically, those covered by insurance plans. In the 1980s the number of private psychiatric hospitals doubled although many state facilities closed (Dorwart and Schlesinger 1988). Partly because mental health costs have risen faster than other medical expenditures, and partly because consumers of psychiatric care have less political leverage than other health care consumers, current proposals for comprehensive health care funding promise to limit mental health coverage by setting arbitrary, yearly limits.

Managed Care and Psychotherapy

Escalating costs have triggered a backlash by third-party payers against providers and the development of a number of cost-control strategies. These include prospective payment plans in which hospitals or other providers receive a predetermined fixed fee for a given episode of illness, capitation plans that limit total outlays for a patient each year, fee schedules, limits on coverage of an episode of illness, and lifetime limits on total mental health costs. Many of these approaches are combined with some sort of managed care oversight that aims to contain current expenditures.

Insurance plans typically have specific limits on coverage for mental disorders. Yet even within those parameters, managed care reviewers typically demand justification to continue care. Denial of payment can readily occur before those limits are reached. In short, mental health providers are forced to justify continuance throughout the course of treatment. Requests for telephone calls at short intervals to obtain authorization and requirements to repeatedly fill out reports serve as subtle inducements to limit the extent of care. Reportedly, mental health providers have been told that their patterns of practice will be monitored and that alleged overuse, regardless of the coverage available to the patient, will have consequences. In preferred provider organizations (PPOs) or independent practice associations (IPAs), that could mean being dropped from the panel of mental health providers (Group for the Advancement of Psychiatry Committee on Therapy 1992).

Managed care has come to exert a profound and increasing influence on the practice of psychiatry, particularly the practice of psychotherapy. It forces the psychotherapist into the position of serving two masters (Levinsky 1984)—the patient and the payer. Often these are at odds with one another, and conflicts ensue that threaten the function and stability of the therapeutic alliance (Sabin 1992). Clinicians are encouraged to prescribe and conduct therapy that they may believe to be inadequate or inappropriate for the patient. Whereas the practitioners of the past struggled against economic temptation, today health care plans embrace and institutionalize economic solutions to conflicts of interest (Group for the Advancement of Psychiatry Committee on Therapy 1992). A few examples illustrate the dilemma for the psychotherapist, including the group psychotherapist.

A patient who presents to a clinician with symptoms of anxiety or depression may be encouraged, through the overseer, to accept a course of pharmacotherapy or short-term cognitive therapy because those are relatively inexpensive. Yet that patient's symptoms could emanate from long-standing conflicts over vocational success or chronic difficulties with intimacy for which long-term individual or group psychotherapy would prove more beneficial. The managed care company, by advocating the less-expensive treatment, will serve the insurance company's needs but not the patient's. Moreover, the cost to society from vocational failure, divorce, and family problems that can affect children are not factored in. Managed care oversight in this instance could cost society more in the long run.

For some patients, crisis intervention and short-term treatments that aim to relieve symptomatic distress may suffice; however, others can be left vulnerable to relapse unless enduring character traits are also attended to. "Conflicts over methods of treatment pose the commonest threats to therapeutic alliance in managed care practice" (Sabin 1992, p. 31).

Patients and managed care companies can unwittingly collaborate, even if they don't have direct contact with one another, to advocate for a treatment plan that is at variance with clinical need. Even though most research reviews have found little outcome differentials between individual and group psychotherapy, patients prefer to have individual treatment (Budman et al. 1988). One can easily imagine situations in which patients and managed care companies would opt for infrequent individual treatment, perhaps with an ad hoc schedule of appointments, rather than weekly group psychotherapy sessions.

Conversely, there could be instances when the clinician and the patient collaborate against the managed care company at the expense of clinical efficacy. The two may focus on realistic problems with "the system" of cost containment and blame it for a gamut of difficulties whose origins are intrapsychic and/or transferential. Both can scapegoat the company to avoid painful affects that belong in treatment.

These examples demonstrate that there are conflicting interests among the three sectors of society involved in mental health care: the health care providers, the patients, and those who pay the costs. Historically, this tripartite system is relatively new. Before the early 1960s, psychotherapy was by and large paid for by patients themselves. Except for the tax deductibility of treatment through which the government partly subsidized psychotherapy, it was a bilateral arrangement between patient and practitioner, usually a psychiatrist. With the extension of health care coverage to mental disorders, third-party reimbursers became part of the equation. As a consequence, psychotherapy, which evolved from a humanistic to a scientific enterprise, is now becoming a corporate one (Karasu 1992). With the shift toward group practice, institutional structures for service delivery, and the introduction of prepaid financing, we are witnessing what has been aptly termed *the industrialization* of mental health care (Bittker 1985).

The demographics of the providers of psychotherapy have changed over the last 30 years. Whereas at one time the typical practitioner was a psychiatrist or perhaps a doctoral-level psychologist, today there are more than 150,000 psychotherapists in this country (Karasu 1992) belonging to various disciplines (e.g., psychology, social work, counseling, nursing) and whose training varies widely. Cost-conscious organizations have taken advantage of this change. HMOs characteristically use lower-cost therapists than does the surrounding community (Manning et al. 1987). Often this gets translated into providers with less training. Here is another instance where economizing can affect the quality of care.

Purchasers of psychotherapy are no longer just patients, but are more often employers who operate through their own negotiations with third-party payers. Proposals for managed competition will further the shift of decision making away from the therapist-patient duo and toward fourth parties. These are entities whose interests are solely economic. They will be constructed for profit, will be accountable to stockholders, and will therefore devise methods for providing passable services for the least amount of expense.

Whereas psychotherapy in its heyday was a caring enterprise, with managed care it has often become an adversarial one. With managed competition, the system of mental health care delivery will have limited capacity to function empathically.

Psychotherapy and Managed Competition

Managed care constitutes micromanagement of health care costs. Reviewers look at each episode of illness to determine where expenditures can be trimmed. There is little effort to consider the expenditures of one episode as a cost savings against future episodes. Likewise, there is no thought given to treatment of one condition (e.g., a psychiatric disorder) as a cost savings against the need for treatment of other conditions (e.g., medical or surgical). Yet that is precisely where psychiatric treatment has proven cost effective. A variety of mental health treatments have been shown to reduce the overall cost of medical care, presumably through reduced utilization (Holder and Blose 1987; Jones and Vischi 1979; Mumford et al. 1984).

Planners of universal health care under managed competition should consider overall costs. So should executives of existing comprehensive health care plans, such as HMOs or other capitation programs. Sometimes they do, but often they don't. Psychological treatments, particularly group psychotherapy, may prove to be economically efficacious in efforts to control health care budgets.

Mumford et al. (1984) performed a meta-analysis of 58 controlled studies and did an analysis of a major insurer's health claim files over a 4-year period. The mental health treatment studies were ones that used a potpourri of short-term interventions. These investigators found that total medical costs rose more slowly over time in the cohort that received the mental health services compared with a control group without such treatment. Cost savings were confined to inpatient charges. Notably, nonpsychiatric inpatient charges showed the greatest reduction for those over age 55. This study not only showed that psychiatric intervention can be cost effective in terms of overall health costs, but it also suggested that the savings are realized more readily with certain categories of care (e.g., hospital costs) and with certain populations. These findings can point the direction for future research on the economizing of health care costs.

Between 1989 and 1992, the Civilian Health and Medical Program of the Uniformed Services (CHAMPUS) increased its yearly outpatient psychiatric expenditures by 28%. This happened when access to outpatient psychotherapy was deliberately eased. The result was a net savings of $200 million, which was twice the outpatient budget. The benefit came from a reduction in psychiatric hospitalization (Gabbard et al. 1993).

Numerous studies have shown the cost effectiveness of psychiatric treatments that serve as alternatives to hospitalization (Sharfstein et al. 1993). Patients with a history of trauma have been shown to be heavy users of medical and surgical care. So are those who have depression. Patients with self-destructive behavior, such as those with depression or borderline conditions, also use emergency rooms more than others. Their symptoms remit and this usage declines after psychotherapy, resulting in savings of emergency care costs (Gabbard et al. 1993). That should encourage HMOs and PPOs to make broader use of psychotherapeutic services to control health costs. Additionally, half of all depressed patients experience functional impairment at work. That observation could encourage corporate insurers to factor into their budgets the benefits accrued when treatment produces a decrease in lost productivity at work.

There are a plethora of outcome studies in the literature comparing individual to group psychotherapy for the treatment of a variety of psychiatric disorders. Meta-analyses of these have consistently shown the two modalities to be equally effective (Orlinsky and Howard 1986; Smith et al. 1980; Tillitski 1990; Toseland and Siporin 1986). But in one instance (Shapiro and Shapiro 1982), individual therapy was found to be slightly more successful. Regardless, since group psychotherapy is less expensive than individual treatment, it is clearly more cost efficient (Dies 1986; Toseland and Siporin 1986). Unfortunately, most comparative studies do not consider discriminate responses according to age and diagnosis and fail to control for the variations of practice. More work needs to be done to evaluate the cost effectiveness of differential therapeutics in order to determine which patient populations are more responsive to different modalities and, within a modality, which of its methods prove superior.

In contrast to studies on the cost-effectiveness of psychiatric treatment in general, little research has been done to evaluate the benefits of group psychotherapy in reducing the overall costs of medical care. There are only two studies on this in the literature. The first (Budman et al. 1982) examined the effects of short-term groups in a private HMO on medical utilization (including visits to nonpsychiatric physicians), laboratory costs, and mental health visits. Severely disturbed patients were excluded, as were those in crisis. The enrollees were generally young, healthy, and well-educated. A significant reduction in overall medical costs (33%) was found. However, this was more than offset by the cost of the group therapy itself. In part, the negative cost-benefit ratio related to the nature of the population sample, because they were infrequent users of medical services to begin with.

In a more recent study, Weiner (1992) used a very different sample and found strikingly different utilization effects. These patients for the most part had both chronic psychiatric problems and multiple, chronic problems of physical health. They were poorly educated and economically disadvantaged. Most were unemployed and some received disability payments. They were treated in a clinic by psychiatric residents in heterogeneous, open-ended groups. The type of psychotherapy was supportive and the focus was pragmatic. The therapists had regular contact with other clinic physicians.

Comparisons were made between overall medical utilization 12 months before starting group therapy and up to 18 months after its initiation. There were no decreases in the use of outpatient medical or psychiatric services. In fact, overall use of psychotropic medication and attendance at medical clinics increased. The increase resulted in part from the efforts of the group therapists to coordinate service delivery and to encourage more regular attendance at other clinics. Yet, increased use of outpatient psychiatric and medical services was more than offset by a decline in psychiatric and nonpsychiatric hospitalizations. The decrease in psychiatric inpatient utilization was far more dramatic than that for medical admissions, and the overall cost savings were considerable. This appeared to be the result of the impact that group psychotherapy had on outpatient treatment compliance, including medication compliance. These results affirm clinical intuition—namely, that programs that engage the sickest and least-functional psychiatric patients are economically sound.

Discussion

Piper aptly notes in Chapter 3 that time-limited group psychotherapy works, at least under research conditions. That has been amply demonstrated in numerous studies (e.g., Orlinsky and Howard 1986). Moreover, as both Piper and MacKenzie state, literature reviews of comparative studies of individual and group psychotherapies attest to their comparable efficacy. The evidence from the research literature argues that group treatment is cost efficient (Dies 1986). Specifically, as Piper notes, it is four times more efficient. Why, then, do not more insurance plans and managed care reviewers encourage the use of group therapy? Many plans cover 20 sessions of psychotherapy per year but invariably fail to differentiate individual from group treatment. Would not it be, as the research evidence demonstrates, cheaper to cover 30 sessions of group psychotherapy rather than 20 of individual treatment? Partial answers to these questions can come from a critical examination of Piper's study of brief treatment for persons who have experienced loss.

As every clinician, knows homogeneous groups produce more rapid relief of symptoms than do heterogeneous groups. That is true even when they fail to influence those personality traits that underlie and contribute to the patient's condition. Third-party payers can be persuaded to support group treatments of Axis I disorders when they are the basis of homogeneous grouping. Examples include eating disorders, somatoform disorder, alcoholism, depression, and so forth. But they are less likely to support treatment when Axis I disorders are not the basis of homogeneity, such as found in groups composed of incest survivors, avoidant personalities, parents of troubled youngsters, the lonely elderly, deprived adolescents, and so on.

When HMOs were new on the scene, health care professionals visualized providing preventive services. Some even offered bereavement counseling. However, by and large these services were sacrificed to cost containment (Group for the Advancement of Psychiatry Committee on Therapy 1992). It is doubtful that managed care systems will continue to pay for treatment of conditions that they consider to be problems of living, not psychiatric disorders. They certainly would not reimburse the cost of the seminar for therapists that was part of the program reported by Piper in Chapter 3. It should be noted that the addition of the seminar cut cost-efficiency in half.

Homogeneous grouping according to patients' circumstances is usually more effective than grouping by diagnosis, although there are some exceptions to this (e.g., eating disorders and alcoholism). Bereaved individuals have more in common with one another (for purposes of psychotherapy) than do, for example, those with dysthymic disorder. Piper's cohort included 11% with a diagnosis of dependent personality disorder and 10% with adjustment disorder, conditions whose treatment managed care would deem nonreimbursable.

Managed care companies consider relief of some specific symptoms worthy of treatment, but not others. For example, in the case of bereavement, they would reimburse for the alleviation of depressive symptoms and improvements in vital areas of social functioning, but would not value improvement in self-esteem or relief from intrusive thoughts about the lost person. They would consider improvement in these latter areas as related to personal well-being and not "medically" significant. Quality assurance reviewers always ask "Is this treatment medically necessary?" but their definition of necessity excludes a substantial portion of patients treated in the studies found in the research literature.

Piper's program is situated at a university hospital that is one of the major triage points in the city for psychiatric patients. In the context of a single-payer system such as in Canada, cost management can consider a variety of medical and social benefits accrued from preventive treatment. Under a system of managed competition, corporate and regional alliances that cover the socially disadvantaged may do the same. In contrast, a system of micromanagement of mental health costs will not take such larger considerations into account.

Piper's program is located at a center that combines research and practice. Outside of academic centers or other large service systems, it is often hard to find a large enough pool of patients to develop treatments that have homogeneous grouping. Additionally, research centers provide certain amenities—such as efforts to solicit patients and special training for therapists—that foster an esprit de corps. Such amenities are not found in ordinary practice, not even in a PPO. This means that findings from research centers are not always transportable to actual practice. If researchers wish to have an impact on managed care as it stands today, they will need to design studies that address the concerns of quality assurance reviewers and that are relevant to ordinary clinical practice.

The program described by Melson in Chapter 6 fits the model of a regional health alliance—that is, an HIPC. It is part of an HMO that has 38,000 enrollees and uses case managers to triage patients. Because of its size, it can develop specialized programs such as the one he describes for treatment of resistant patients who have associated personality disorders and significant functional impairments. The latter is an important factor. These patients have repeated inpatient admissions and multiple emergency room visits, are suicide risks, and are frequent users of other medical services. Programs that select patients whose psychiatric treatment yields a net medical cost offset through reduction of other medical expenditures have appeal to large provider networks. The benefit that Melson's program had in reducing days lost from work might only appeal to an employer-based provider. To an unaffiliated HMO, that would be a marginal benefit.

Creating large organizations for the delivery of care has its downside. A recent nationwide study of more than 17,000 patients (Rubin et al. 1993) found widespread dissatisfaction with HMOs. In contrast, patients who saw independent physicians felt that their doctors were easier to reach by telephone, more available for visits, showed more interest in their well-being, and provided better explanations of their treatment. In short, in HMOs there was a lower level of customer (patient) satisfaction. Previous studies have shown that patients who are satisfied with their doctors are more likely to return for further care. Large, impersonal systems of care by their very nature discourage use of services. There is a clear danger that the triage process in managed care settings will result in patients bouncing around the system without continuity of care. Quality of care goes down whenever systemic forces serve to dampen the use and delivery of services.

When approving a course of therapy, today managed care reviewers generally inquire into four areas of treatment: 1) whether the condition being treated is covered by the insurance contract; 2) whether the treatment plan is a customary one for that condition; 3) whether the patient is making progress with treatment; and 4) how long treatment will take (Allen 1988). Identification of the condition is based on DSM-III-R (American Psychiatric Association 1987). Regrettably, as MacKenzie notes in Chapter 1, for Axis II personality disorders the DSM-III-R categorical system is unsatisfactory. There is considerable overlap between entities, its nosology is not very relevant to clinical practice, some of its terminology rests on uncertain foundation, and it is descriptive and arbitrarily excludes observations derived from psychodynamic investigation (Kernberg 1984).

As MacKenzie also notes in Chapter 1, there is no difference between the personality dimensions of the major disorders and those of the general population. In fact, clinical relevance lies in the level of dysfunction that results from maladaptive use of personality rather than in absolute diagnosis. A system of categorization based on levels of dysfunction may prove more useful to health care planners in delineating criteria for reimbursement by third-party payers. In the past, research has dictated nosology; in the future, reimbursement could.

It is unclear whether managed competition will provide treatment that has a beneficial impact on the quality of life unless its economic benefits can also be demonstrated. Managed care providers have up to now been loath to pay for treatments that enhance the quality of life, which they narrowly define as "problems in living." In other words, they do not pay for psychological pain unless there are accompanying major psychiatric symptoms. Yet in other branches of medicine they do pay for psychological pain; for example, they pay for orthopedic injuries that affect the quality of life. The psychiatric profession has yet to establish a corresponding principle of payment for treatment that relieves pain. In the last analysis, this applies to a gamut of personality traits and disorders. Consider the following example:

> A 38-year-old man with a diagnosis of bipolar disorder had three brief hospitalizations over a 2-year period. The first was the result of a full-blown manic episode; however, the last two, which were preceded by a recurrence of mania, were precipitated by purposeful discontinuation of lithium. At the time of the second hospitalization, the patient fabricated some history and told a new treating psychiatrist that the former one had advised him to stop the medication, which was a lie.
>
> Before the first manic episode, this patient had a history of severe interpersonal problems. He had been argumentative with co-workers and supervisors. As a result, he was fired from several jobs. His marriage of 5 years had ended in divorce 8 years previously because his wife had found him to be insufferably arrogant, demanding, and callous. The diagnoses were Axis I bipolar disorder and Axis II narcissistic personality disorder.
>
> The patient's managed care provider agreed to pay for outpatient treatment of the personality disorder only because they were convinced that it was the underlying factor in medication noncompliance. But would they have paid for psychotherapy before this patient had ever had a manic episode, when his pathology was manifested merely by work and social problems? That is doubtful.

Reviewers are in a position to place restrictions on the clinician's freedom to prescribe the best mode of treatment. Even though first-line managed care reviewers supposedly merely act as advisers, they have increasingly exerted leverage over clinical practice. This is because the final decision to pay or not to pay (e.g., for the psychotherapy) is made by the company. Although most health care contracts allow for an appeal process, the final determination as to what is "medically necessary" is made by the company's medical director, not by the practitioner.

Frequently, reviewers disallow procedures that are not the norm in clinical practice, such as a family session and a group session on the same day. They place limitations on the use of innovative methods such as marathon sessions. Reviewers are also likely to deny payment for standard procedures that seem to them to involve a duplication of services; for example, the use of combined individual and group psychotherapy.

The result of this type of review may be to restrict the freedom to vary practice according to clinical need, to inhibit innovation, and to deter experimentation with new approaches (Allen 1979). Managed care oversight at its worst, because of fear engendered of possible breaches of confidentiality, threatens to interdict the treatment of certain people who worry about exposure, such as paranoid patients, those involved in divorce cases or other legal proceedings, and those in positions that are publicly visible (Allen 1979).

Stone in Chapter 7 and Cross in Chapter 2 both outlined some of the factors that affect clinical work when operating in a managed care setting. Cross particularly described the organization of group psychotherapy programming. However, managed care is not necessarily the same as managed competition. If the Jackson Hole Group wins the day, this volume may need to be revised.

The program at the Mayo Clinic described by Peterson in Chapter 5 is unique in three ways. First, it is an intensive, 3-week day treatment program. However, it is one with an unusual emphasis on psychotherapy, specifically group psychotherapy. Second, it is populated by a preponderance of patients with somatoform and depressive disorders. Lastly, insurance carriers had given precertification approval. Closer examination demonstrates how unusual it is to get preapproval for such innovative treatment. By and large, these patients carried diagnoses within the neurotic spectrum of disorders and most of them were dysthymic.

Ordinarily, managed care providers would not pay for such an expensive treatment program for these patients, but would opt for the use of a combination of pharmacotherapy and supportive psychotherapy. That approach, which is cost effective in the short run, as Peterson notes, may deprive large numbers of patients of a therapeutic experience that could have a lasting beneficial impact on their lives. In this case, the managed care reviewers were probably accommodating for two reasons. First, the program was located at a prestigious medical center whose affiliation seemed suited to the treatment of such patients who present predominantly with somatic symptoms, if not a frank somatoform disorder. Second, these patients had failed to be helped by previous treatments and were proven to be treatment resistant.

Will managed care continue to pay for this treatment? That is a question yet to be answered. The patients showed decided improvement that persisted at 8 months follow-up. These results are heartening from a psychiatric perspective, but what do they mean from an economic standpoint? More specifically, will this intensive psychotherapy program produce an offset of medical costs? That is a crucial financial question.

The patients described by Rice in Chapter 4, who were treated at a large community mental health center, were also high users of medical and mental health services. In addition to having chronic depressive symptoms, they were quite dysfunctional. They had limited financial and personal resources and were subject to chronic psychosocial stress. They are typical of patients treated in the public sector. So were those in the program described by Stone in Chapter 7, where chronic patients with personality and anxiety disorders were maintained successfully with group treatment. Regrettably, current proposals for comprehensive universal health care promise to limit psychiatric coverage, which will, in effect, exclude those requiring chronic care; this is shortsighted.

Approximately 5 million Americans have severe mental disorders. Treatment now costs the country an estimated $20 billion a year in direct health costs. When social costs are added to this figure, the toll approaches $74 billion. The increase comes from estimates of costs incurred from lost productivity, use of the social service and criminal justice systems, and use of other health care services (American Psychiatric Association 1993). These costs are now borne by the general health care system and by society at large. Given the solid body of research evidence that treatment for severe mental disorders is effective, limiting access to such treatment is penny-wise and pound-foolish. Helping these individuals to function more productively would benefit the country, both socially and financially. But convincing the nation's politicians and financial planners of that is extremely doubtful.

Training in the Future

Although the leaders of academic psychiatry are in agreement that training in psychotherapy is essential to the future of psychiatry, the actual time allotted for that task in residency programs is shrinking (Tasman and Kay 1987). Today, the average resident gets minimal exposure to psychodynamic psychotherapy. This has prompted a joint task force of the American Association of Directors of Psychiatry Residency Training and the Association for Academic Psychiatry to propose that a minimum curriculum be mandated (Mohl et al. 1990) that would include training in expressive psychotherapy.

Practicing psychodynamic psychotherapy forces the psychiatrist to observe, analyze, and try to understand complex interactive forces within people; to examine the effect of unconscious mental functioning on normal and pathological relationships; and to observe the vicissitudes of psychopathology over time. Training in individual psychotherapy helps the resident to learn about these phenomena from an intrapsychic perspective. Training in group psychotherapy does the same from an interpersonal one. That has educational value even if the trainee does not practice psychotherapy later on in his or her career. Many will not, given the trends in the field. It can be anticipated that treatment decisions will be increasingly influenced by fiscal considerations, resulting in preferences for low-cost services such as crisis intervention, time-limited, and symptom-focused treatments (Group for the Advancement of Psychiatry Committee on Therapy 1992).

Government policies that encourage a decrease of specialization in medicine and the training of more primary care providers may, because of shifting resources, change the role of the psychiatrist of the future. The Department of Health and Human Services has encouraged the development of clinical practice guidelines for a variety of medical conditions (Rush 1993). Guidelines for psychiatric disorders are being developed and a few have been published. These will enable primary care physicians and nonpsychiatric mental health providers to treat many patients with uncomplicated disorders. As a result, psychiatrists in the future may see and treat only the more complex patient cases. Yet they will still have the major role in strategic planning of service delivery and will continue to oversee and supervise those who conduct psychotherapy.

In order to meet the demands of the future, psychiatrists will still have to be experts in the management of treatment relationships as they are influenced by transference. Psychiatrists will need to know how the group dynamics of service delivery systems influence the effectiveness of treatment. Thus, training in psychodynamic psychotherapy, including group psychotherapy, will prove invaluable.

Training in the future should include the study of the sociology of psychotherapy. All too frequently, psychotherapists working in managed care and prepaid systems are ignorant of organizational constraints and are not adept at integrating institutional factors into the treatment. Ideally, large systems that deliver care should take advantage of the multiple skills of its practitioners so that patients can be offered finely tuned prescriptions for care. That would enable patients to receive different treatments at different points in their recovery. For example, a specific patient may require pharmacotherapy at one time, cognitive therapy at another, and group psychotherapy at still a third juncture. The Residency Review Committee of the American Psychiatric Association has begun to address this problem. Its latest guidelines on training require that residents now have at least some training in patterns of delivery of psychiatric services (e.g., HMOs, PPOs) and in managed care (Accreditation Council for Graduate Medical Education 1993). A recent informal survey of resident leaders showed that formal training in managed care is sorely lacking (Scully 1993).

In the future, residency programs will need to educate trainees about how economically driven decisions affect patient care, how to deal with managed care reviewers whenever they are in disagreement, and how to respond ethically when there are conflicts between standards for care and their own economic interests. Thus, although training in psychodynamic psychotherapy and group dynamics should continue to be part of psychiatric residency programs in the next century, the education of future clinicians should integrate a knowledge of sociology. How that will be done is yet to be determined. Perhaps a new generation of leaders in education will span what are now separate disciplines. Perhaps there will be medical sociologists or sociological psychiatrists to guide the way.

References

Accreditation Council for Graduate Medical Education (ACGME): Revision of Special Requirements for Psychiatry. Accreditation Council for Graduate Medical Education, Chicago, Memorandum of July 7, 1993

Allen MG: Peer review of group therapy: Washington, DC, 1972–1977. Am J Psychiatry 136:444–447, 1979

Allen MG: Psychiatric peer review: a current perspective. Psychiatric Annals 18:487–491, 1988

American Psychiatric Association: Diagnostic and Statistical Manual of Mental Disorders, 3rd Edition, Revised. Washington, DC, American Psychiatric Association, 1987

American Psychiatric Association: Health care reform for Americans with severe mental illnesses: report of the National Advisory Mental Health Council. Am J Psychiatry 150:1447–1465, 1993

Bittker TE: The industrialization of American psychiatry. Am J Psychiatry 142:149–154, 1985

Budman SH, Demby A, Randal M: Psychotherapeutic outcome and reduction in medical utilization: a cautionary tale. Professional Psychology 13:200–207, 1982

Budman SH, Demby A, Redondo JP, et al: Comparative outcome in time-limited individual and group psychotherapy. Int J Group Psychother 38:63–86, 1988

Dies RR: Practical, theoretical, and empirical foundations for group psychotherapy, in Psychiatry Update: American Psychiatric Association Annual Review, Vol 5. Edited by Frances AJ, Hales RE. Washington, DC, American Psychiatric Press, 1986, pp 659–677

Dorwart RA, Schlesinger M: Privatization of psychiatric services. Am J Psychiatry 145:543–553, 1988

Einthoven A, Kronick R: A consumer-choice health plan for the 1990s: universal health insurance in a system designed to promote quality and economy. N Engl J Med 320:29–37, 1989

Gabbard GO, Lazar SG, Hersh EK: Cost-offset studies show value of psychotherapy. Psychiatric Times 10(8):21, 1993

Grinfeld MJ: Are we close to national health care reform? Psychiatric Times 10(6):56–57, 1993

Group for the Advancement of Psychiatry (GAP) Committee on Therapy: Report #133: Psychotherapy in the Future. Group for the Advancement of Psychiatry, Washington, DC, American Psychiatric Press, 1992

Health Care Financing Administration: Cumulative growth in Gross National Product and National Health Expenditures, 1980–2000. Washington, DC, Health Care Financing Administration, 1991

Holder AD, Blose JO: Changes in health care costs and utilization associated with mental health treatment. Hosp Community Psychiatry 38:1070–1075, 1987

Jones KR, Vischi TR: Impact of alcohol, drug abuse and mental health treatment on medical care utilization. Med Care 17 (suppl 12):1–82, 1979

Karasu TB: The worst of times, the best of times: psychotherapy in the 1990s. Journal of Psychotherapy Practice and Research 1:2–15, 1992

Kernberg OF: Severe Personality Disorders: Psychotherapeutic Strategies. New Haven, CT, Yale University Press, 1984

Levinsky N: The physician's master. N Engl J Med 311:1573–1575, 1984

Manning AG, Wells KB, Benjamin B: Use of outpatient mental health services over time in a health maintenance organization and fee-for-service plans. Am J Psychiatry 144:283–287, 1987

Marmor TR: Making sense of the national health care debate. Paper presented at the 146th annual meeting of the American Psychiatric Association, San Francisco, CA, May 1993

Mirin SM: The changing face of mental health care: doing what's needed, doing what's right. Psychiatric Times 10(7):29–31, 1993

Mohl PC, Lomax J, Tasman A, et al: Psychotherapy training for the psychiatrist of the future. Am J Psychiatry 147:7–13, 1990

Mumford E, Schlesinger HJ, Glass GV, et al: A new look at evidence about reduced cost of medical utilization following mental health treatment. Am J Psychiatry 141:1145–1158, 1984

Orlinsky DE, Howard KI: Process and outcome in psychotherapy, in Handbook of Psychotherapy and Behavior Change, 3rd Edition. Edited by Garfield SL, Bergin AE. New York, Wiley, 1986, pp 311–381

Rubin HR, Gandek MS, Rogers WH, et al: Patients' ratings of outpatient visits in different practice settings. JAMA 270:835–840, 1993

Rush AJ: Clinical practice guidelines: good news, bad news, or no news? Arch Gen Psychiatry 50:483–490, 1993

Sabin JE: The therapeutic alliance in managed care mental health practice. Journal of Psychotherapy Practice and Research 1:29–36, 1992

Scully JH: Residents' education and managed care. Psychiatric Residents' Newsletter 18(2):1–2, 1993

Shapiro DA, Shapiro D: Meta-analysis of comparative therapy outcome studies: a replication and refinement. Psychol Bull 92:581–604, 1982

Sharfstein SS, Stoline AM, Goldman HH: Psychiatric care and health insurance reform. Am J Psychiatry 150:7–18, 1993

Smith ML, Glass GV, Miller TI: The Benefits of Psychotherapy. Baltimore, MD, Johns Hopkins University Press, 1980

Tasman A, Kay J: Setting the stage: residency training in 1986, in Training Psychiatrists for the 90s: Issues and Recommendations. Edited by Nadelson CC, Robinowitz CB. Washington, DC, American Psychiatric Press, 1987, pp 49–59

Tillitski CJ: A meta-analysis of estimated effect sizes for group vs. individual vs. control treatments. Int J Group Psychother 40:215–224, 1990

Toseland RW, Siporin M: When to recommend group treatment: a review of the clinical and the research literature. Int J Group Psychother 36:171–201, 1986

Weiner MF: Group therapy reduces medical and psychiatric hospitalization. Int J Group Psychother 42:267–275, 1992

Index

*Page numbers printed in **boldface** type refer to tables or figures.*